Quit Smoking

The Most Effective Method to Quit Smoking

(The Easy Escape From Nicotine Dependance to Restore Your Health)

Willie Bounds

Published By **Jackson Denver**

Willie Bounds

All Rights Reserved

Quit Smoking: The Most Effective Method to Quit Smoking (The Easy Escape From Nicotine Dependance to Restore Your Health)

ISBN 978-1-77485-549-2

No part of this guidebook shall be reproduced in any form without permission in writing from the publisher except in the case of brief quotations embodied in critical articles or reviews.

Legal & Disclaimer

The information contained in this ebook is not designed to replace or take the place of any form of medicine or professional medical advice. The information in this ebook has been provided for educational & entertainment purposes only.

The information contained in this book has been compiled from sources deemed reliable, and it is accurate to the best of the Author's knowledge; however, the Author cannot guarantee its accuracy and validity and cannot be held liable for any errors or omissions. Changes are periodically made to this book. You must consult your doctor or get professional medical advice before using any of the suggested remedies, techniques, or information in this book.

Upon using the information contained in this book, you agree to hold harmless the Author from and against any damages, costs, and expenses, including any legal fees potentially resulting from the application of any of the information provided by this guide. This disclaimer applies to any damages or injury caused by the use and application, whether directly or indirectly, of any advice or information presented, whether for breach of contract, tort, negligence, personal injury, criminal intent, or under any other cause of action.

You agree to accept all risks of using the information presented inside this book. You need to consult a professional medical practitioner in order to ensure you are both able and healthy enough to participate in this program.

Table of contents

INTRODUCTION 1

CHAPTER 1: THE PREMISES AND THE BASICS..... 13

CHAPTER 2: BEGINNING OF CHANGING YOUR MIND. 27

CHAPTER 3: WHAT'S TO COME AND THE BEST TOOLS TO HELP YOU ON YOUR JOURNEY.......... 42

CHAPTER 4: DETERMINATION 86

CHAPTER 5: CONSCIOUSNESS AND UNCONSCIOUS ALIGNMENT 95

CHAPTER 6: DAY ZERO 106

CHAPTER 7: ILLUSION OF SMOKING CIGARETTES 116

CHAPTER 8: WHY DOES SMOKING SEEM SO DIFFICULT TO STOP? 124

CHAPTER 9: A EMOTIONAL PUSH 130

CHAPTER 10: PSYCHOLOGICAL BARRIERS 132

CHAPTER 11: WHAT'S THE SCIENCE BEHIND BAD HABITS.. 139

CHAPTER 12: WHAT CAN I STOP SMOKING 143

CHAPTER 13: WHAT BROUGHT YOU TO SMOKING?... 149

CONCLUSIONS 182

Introduction
The process of improving your life is never simple, and changes like eating healthier, exercising more, and so on. You must overcome the resistance of the lifestyle that you want to break away from breaking the habits requires some energy, concentration and effort However, if you manage to stay consistent and committed, eventually you will get more momentum, and as you advance, things will become simpler and more straightforward until you can live in an better life.

I wish I could tell you that overcoming an addiction comes with a and difficult hurdle to conquer however, the reality, as you will see when you read this article, it isn't the same. Having an addiction raises the bar to a new height it is a fight you'll face with yourself, your emotions, which as we'll discover in the future, they are the ones who decide the human behaviour, therefore you have to test yourself against yourself as well as your own personal wishes and desires, your paradigms, basic instincts, and hope to succeed. This is far more than taking yourself out of your comfort zone since it is merely a way to making healthier choices like eating healthier or exercising.

The dangers of addiction should not be taken lightly. They can ruin you and take everything including your possessions and material things, to your job, family, as well as your self-image and respect. They can destroy your life on many different ways and levels. Addictions are truely invisible creatures that remain at the forefront of our minds they manipulate us like puppets. To defeat them requires a plan that is disciplined, determined, and a strong drive to get away from them. I'll share the blue print that I could use to build on my plan of action and successfully overcoming this destructive habit. The other elements (will force, drive,, etc.) will be provided by you.

Like any recipe for cooking is, you will need the necessary steps, your ingredients to use and the determination to get yourself into the process of preparing the ingredients according to the method the recipe instructs you to prepare your food. If you don't possess the ingredients, recipe or the desire to get yourself involved it is likely that you won't be able to be able to cook a meal.

To know that you've got what it takes to be successful and succeed, consider how much are you willing to go I was in despair, and I tried and failed numerous times with disappointing failures frustrated and anger, despair, etc. My efforts included special products specifically designed be used for this purpose however there was no way to make it work. I was terribly depressed and felt helpless. If you're in the middle of the same place then you're at the right place to begin.

Notepads are essential You will require it whenever you read something of value note it down rather than just mark them up, the effect on your brain is different and you'll also have a step-by-step roadmap once you've gone through the reading process.

Through this guide, I'll give you a plan that will help you eliminate bad habits. Although I can't guarantee that success. But it is sure that if you adhere to the program and resolve to follow the steps is highly likely that you will be able to overcome it and attain your goal.

The main subject of this article is tobacco, as it was one of the things I was fighting against and the reason behind it is that I was able to get rid of the habit of smoking with the information you'll discover here. That does doesn't mean you can't make use of this method for other goals, in the end of the day, we're facing the same issue but with different substances. The issue of attachment to a dangerous and powerful addiction substance is within the mind. You are able to connect it to any substance if you adhere to the guidelines outlined in this article although the intensity of dependence between substances is differs, cigarettes are certainly one of the strongest. So in the event that this method worked for me I am confident that you can apply this battle with success.

It is possible to make an emotional leap to the specific situation you're fighting since, in the end, I believe you'll be able to relate to my experience and what my experiences. I recommend that you search for data relevant to your particular case. i.e. when I mention anything that is related to tobacco in the context of facts. I would encourage you to look into what could apply to your situation.

The method suggested by this book is performed by the mind, and where the causes are stimulated, to result in desired results (i.e. the law of cause and impact) In the end of the day, addictions are what we'll treat. Therefore no matter what you're trying combat, follow the same method, and modify it if needed and then adapt the method to tailor it to your specific needs. In certain instances, I'll be referring to substances that are different than tobacco, but that won't be the case always the case.

As we'll see in the future, the arrangement of a habit within the mind is difficult to overcome because we have a tendency to focusing on things that are tangible. We are able to easily connect with the things we see, combat them them, arrange them, etc. But in the mind, it is something completely different since we are blind in various ways, and we must pay attention to areas that we cannot see which is why the process of forming habits difficult.

When you observe the room is cluttered quickly with quick glances with your eyes you can determine what to do, and it's extremely easy to determine the cause. What happens when you're dealing with a mess in a room you aren't able to perceive? This isn't easy, right? This is why it's so difficult to get rid of our habits. We don't know how to begin, and when you aren't sure of exactly what you're doing and what you are doing, it is difficult to anticipate positive results that keep you motivated. frequently, you'll feel sadness, despair, and similar feelings like I felt.

To combat this issue (at the very least, for tobacco) we look for and test devices that are tangible, e.g. nicotine gum, e-cigarettes and so on. since that's what we're programmed to do. This is the "normal behaviour" when we consider how we are taught to think and behave in a way that is always based on tangible objects but are they really beneficial? They weren't for me.

It can be a bit complex, however we should apply the same logic that you use when playing an audio track wirelessly via an android phone that is connected to a remote speaker. you are aware that changing an album will require contact with the phone, not the speaker that emits the sound. The same principle applies here, recognizing that the issue lies in the mind. There is the primary goal that will be the primary goal, any other efforts will not be able to aid you, unless they indirectly operate with your brain.

The majority of times, the issue does not have to do with one particular habit. I'm not referring only to harmful behaviors, but as that mind-based problems are rooted in the mind It is likely that you have other things that you're hooked on or habits you wish to eliminate If this is the situation, concentrate only on one habit at a time. A change in habit demands a lot of attention at the beginning stages, similar to like a rocket is burning the most of its fuel to overcome inertia and stay back on track, since once in orbit, it is able to burn off fuel as it is able to continue, but only to adjust or change direction however the major step is initiated at the beginning, as you initiate the cause to create the effect. breaking through the resistance in your mind is equally difficult to do, so take a step-by- method, polishing angles by angles your character like a jeweler who works with diamonds, one step at a at a time. There is lots of time continue learning the new habits that will benefit you in the long run so let's not diminish your chances of success trying to do multiple things at the same simultaneously.

Many thousands of chemical compounds that are harmful for the human body are in cigarettes, the same is true to other addictions. I'm not sure there's one study that has endorsed any positive effects on the body as a result of cigarettes, in fact Any study you discover in this area suggests the same thing and that's why the level of quality of life decreases and the risk of developing diseases could end in the early stages of your life.

It is crucial to keep your eyes open And the greater you learn about the effects of smoking tobacco (or any other chemically toxic substance you became addicted to) the better, as having a clear picture of what your future holds and will boost your motivation to lead a healthier life style and adopt new practices to improve your quality of life. The opening of your eyes experience will be a part of the process since even though you are aware of the facts, studying these facts more deeply will result in an awakening that will help you make a decision. This is a great place to start writing in your notepad.

The more you are able to incorporate numbers and facts into the future, your life, you will have an experience unlike any other that comes from understanding the surface of the facts. At the conclusion of the day you will see that the sole "benefit" is immediate , short moment pleasure and pleasure that is a brief good or tranquil feeling, however at the cost of the most expensive price for it. And I'm in no way talking about cash. Certainly smoking cigarettes is a drain on your pocket and there is no doubt about it However, the actual cost is the reduction in how you live your life in order to lower your life expectancy and your teeth, as well as your well-being, and even your ability to safely climb stairs no matter how basic it may seem.

The more you can open your eyes to the world, the more simple it will be to look up testimonials and attentively listen to them.

I'm certain they'll assist you in making a lasting impression on yourself. You must come to reality and stop being at a loss from the charms created by this drug you're dependent on.

What price would you be willing to sell the day of your life for? Consider for a moment that I had the power to buy your life and include it in mine. What is your price? Take a look! The issue with addiction is that we have lost all awareness of the implications of falling prey to addictions, but for other substances the consequences could be greater, leading to the end of your career broken homes, broken relationships and self-esteem and career, job, and so on. This is what happens when you drink alcohol, for instance. However, the goal isn't to make you feel depressed before we begin the process, but rather an indication of the potential damage you could cause yourself. I'm not going discuss this subject further however it can aid in identifying the negative aspects in the near future. might be ahead if you don't take the right direction and take appropriate actions to improve your situation.

The decision to stop smoking is among the most difficult things that I have ever done. Only someone who has gone through this process will understand how challenging it is even for those who have never had a smoking habit in their life. it may seem simple, however the reality is that being addicted, however it is, can be a bit complicated and is something that you are a dependent on because it has influence over you. To stop the destructive habits associated with brain chemicals like nicotine isn't the same thing as to break an old habit that is not linked to the chemical substance that your body craves. In any event, I'll explain my experience everything to my best abilities how to do it step-by-step so you will benefit by following the same method I did, with a particular focus on the significance of each step, as it can change the game.

If you're a person with this issue on an extensive way and have attempted to stop smoking but had little success for a few months I am sure that these words were written for you. specifically, I am referring to smokers who have smoked around an hour a day and who tried a variety of other methods like nicotine gum patches, e-cigarettes and so on. If you aren't rooted in the habit, I'm not certain if this approach can help. I'm talking about people who smoke on weekends or at social gatherings who smoke when they are drinking, as well as those who smoke a couple of cigarettes a day during the afternoon or the evening, however since it is built on psychological principles I'm sure it might be an option for those of you who are also struggling or at least try the option a go, because since the goal is to enhance your life and smoking is clearly not helping in any way.

Chapter 1: The Premises And The Basics

The best way to begin is to be able to show the complete determination to reach this goal. In fact, this issue is so important that a whole section will be dedicated to it. The majority of people just say that they love smoking, and they do it because they are motivated to keep doing it, which is why they remain smokers. Being a non-smoker and a an addict in the past, I know that the majority of people believe that to avoid admitting failure of failing to quit in the first place, and also to hide that it is more powerful than them, and in the secret, they've failed a number of times. I've used this excuse often when I received an answer whether people are keen to stop or not, they claim they're not interested due to the fact that they enjoy smoking so much. However, when I ask them to be honest by presenting this rationale and they admit that they tried several times to stop but failed.

It's what I refer to as the effect of big walls that occurs when they bond in a cell that has big walls, but no ceiling. climbing a scape is possible , but they view the walls to be so high that after a time they stop trying to climbing anymore. They simply stop trying and declare "I feel at ease here, nothing to worry about and I'll just remain" But what if they were aware that digging in the cell's corner six feet deep, they would discover an entrance key, and could leave at any time If they did, would they still claim they're comfortable and want to remain there? I doubt it. If redemption is extremely difficult, it is overwhelming. However, when we realize there's an opportunity that we believe to be plausible, we take it. This can be seen in those who are stuck in relationships, poor jobs, etc.

A large number of people are "not prepared" to give up, as often I suggest to people a way to stop without patches or any other supplement that is not their own and sometimes they aren't even willing to listen. the addiction is so powerful in their minds and bodies that they are not even willing to a different treatment for their issue It is evident in their eyes. They appear to be in shock when they hear that a different path is available to them. They're terrified and cannot imagine their lives changing in the end, I be aware of that, but I know that the fear is embedded in their minds as a factor in the problem because it completely controls them and, unfortunately, I'm unable to provide a solution to these individuals, it is impossible to help those who aren't willing to accept your assistance, until they reach a point in which they're determined to be free, and regardless of what solution you propose to them, they will not accept it, and if that's your case, the advice I've provided in this article won't help you in any way.

Do you think about that? Consider it for while, imagine somebody who is so deeply into something that they won't even want to listen to you. this can be extended to other scenarios, like toxic relationships in which they isn't willing to part with their spouse, but you won't be at peace if you're emotionally connected to something or someone that is chemical substances like nicotine or alcohol, a person or something else you want to call it.

To lead a life worth living in complete freedom, you must have complete control over your thoughts. to stray from this principle to enjoy some short-term reward from pleasure is acceptable at times I think it's part of the human condition but the control should be exercised throughout the day over your mind. You could even allow this thought to play while you think about it and come to this conclusion on your own. I would suggest that you pause your reading, put aside smoking (or any other addiction) issue, and allow yourself time to consider this before continuing since if you are able to comprehend and work to achieve this goal of controlling your mind, you'll not only be able to get rid of the issue you're here to solve, but will also assist in improving your life above the initial purpose that brought you here.

In re-examining the concept, I realize that those who do not even bother to look to the solution grasp the larger picture. They only listen to their internal voices calling for nicotine, yet they aren't aware of themselves facing a concerned doctor who is looking for the right words to inform them that they've developed some form of cancer that is linked to smokingcigarettes, emphysema or any other ailment that is catastrophic They don't envision themselves with a needle in their arm to administer chemotherapy, or lying in an hospital bed equipped with a device that is able to breathe for them. This should be a nightmare and I hope you weren't part of this group of unfortunates.

If you're at the point of not considering a possible solution due to the fact that it scares you to know that you will not get the amount of nicotine the body requires so you're uninterested in any solution, then that this approach is not likely to help you. however, if you're sick of trying, been crying in your home because you tried and failed as I have done at times, are scared and hopeless, yet you are determined and you haven't discovered the ideal method to free yourself in the foreseeable future, then, my friend I believe that you're on the right place you are reading this. Since that's exactly the way I felt. But I'm getting ahead of myself. I will allow you to read about my experience in the future.

The good news is that people who have been open to listening and trying this with the right chance and confidence they have all had the desired results however, one note of caution there are those who have relapsed after a few months have gone by The main reason for this is that they believed they had a handle on the habit, but eventually they wanted to limit themselves to "social smokers" not a good idea.

This is extremely risky illusion that could get you hooked in the first place Be aware of this should you be successful later on, don't look back. If nicotine (or any other substance you became addicted to) held you captive and you became addicted , it's because you lost control of the substance, and if it happened once and it didn't work, there's no reason why it shouldn't be able to repeat the same thing. Addictive substances can be seductive to your body. You must practice discipline when you get over the fence.

The individuals I am talking about failed their goals of becoming social smokers, and then experienced the same level of devastation like they were in the beginning in the first place. I am going to tell you that it isn't easy to complete the detox process. It is a real challenge, there does not come with butterflies and rainbows You will be reading about issues and experiences I have experienced during my own experience. continuing through this process is not something I am going to do take a step back and do something for yourself, and if you do decide to go through this process and get an end to your habit to quit, you must do so for good. I stopped smoking about 15 years in the past, and it is a blessing that the tobacco smell present is very unpleasant It is a fact that smoking cigarettes is the most stupid thing I've done in my life . I will never smoke again I'm sure you share the same attitude and purpose, as when you are looking to switch from a smoker who is heavy to a smoking with friends, even by this approach you're in the wrong place. In any case, I would like to believe that this message popped up at you is because you're looking for answers and if that is the case, I'm sure you'll get the answers you've been looking for.

The foundation of what I'm going to discuss with you is, as I have already said, an emotional scheme that I believe is the main basis for why this strategy is effective or at the very least works for me. Smoking affects the chemical balance of your brain however only by self-control can you make yourself conform to this. I believe this is the case for those with eating disorders who tend to weigh a lot above or below the amount they should and if this is your case and you choose to follow the same method for both, I'd encourage you to try it but I would not recommend doing both at once take it step by step in the same manner as I have suggested previously and focus on just only one thing at a moment, the reason being that you'll gain control over certain aspects, but you will lose some control temporarily over other things like your temper because of the absence of the addictive substance within your body. This can result in unintentional behaviors because of an imbalance in your brain's chemical levels and, if you're determined to completely make a fresh start in just only a few days to eliminate the two or more habits that you're most likely to fail. require a laser-like focus on the issue and focus tends to diminish when more issues focus your concentration.

This psychological adjustment can seem like turning several knobs in your head in the absence of an appropriate term, however I believe you'll be able to appreciate the final result and this is the reason why you should remain patient, determined and determined. This isn't something you can do in one day. When you're dealing with your mind. adjustments are more like navigating a huge cruise ship. You're turning the steering wheel, and it will take a while before you can actually feel the ship's motion unlike an automobile where it is instantly felt and therefore, it will take a few months to be needed to complete the changes, so don't lose this concept from your mind be aware this is an activity that takes time , and you will not notice results immediately, just like when you eat healthily this morning and then sit up in the mirror, you will not appear slim. It will require time and lots of nutritious meals in order to detoxify and nourish your body in order to rid it of toxins and fats and eventually, you'll look in the mirror and be thinking, I appear slim! Get the short-term reward notion away from your thoughts it will help you in a variety of areas of your life. shorter-term rewards are not useful in general.

It's for your own benefit Once you've reached this point in your life, you'll be able to appreciate what you've left behind. It's hard to appreciate the beauty of things when you're in the middle of the ravages of a storm, but once you make it to the summit of a mountain, you will see how gorgeous the scenery was and is, you're no longer exhausted and realize that the effort to climb were well-worth it. That's how I felt. And once you're at that point all that goes through your mind is why you didn't take the time to do this earlier. I believe you will reach the same level and experience the benefits of living a "free lifestyle". I am aware of the harm I did to myself, however I'm also grateful that the days of my life are over for good.

Smoking cigarettes is a habit which manages to lure you, without adding worth to you in any way. it's absurd from every perspective like I said earlier. the short-term rewards that are accompanied by tangible goods are not the best choice for you. I'm not referring to food in particular, or the healthiest one at the very least and I'm certain there are some exceptions to this rule however, if you look at it from a different perspective an enjoyable, moderately lasting enjoyment is far more significant than a high-pitch, short-term reward. It's simple that we choose more of the latter because of our insufficient discipline, but this is contingent on the level of maturity of the individual and those who have have learned from their mistakes generally prefer the opposite way and this choice is often done with discipline and maturity following a process of thinking has been completed. The behavior to spend money an straightforward example to illustrate the point. Children who are reckless people generally will spend any amount that is available and believe that the reward is short-term is a good thing, whereas people who are older and more mature have more fun saving money and feel the satisfaction of security knowing they have savings available I would consider this as a long-lasting pleasureand consider the spending as a reward of a high-pitch of buying something enjoyable that brings excitement for a brief period of time.

A word of caution must be made at this point. Please be sure to read the entire article before beginning. This isn't something you have to read for two pages, then continue to work on them until you go through further steps to then follow the steps, or in the same way it's not a recipe for cooking which you follow step-by-step while you read and follow the instructions in the document taking it step-by-step it is than a recipe that needs to be go through in detail, fully comprehend the concept, comprehend the concept, and be prepared for the beginning and then start off. I will describe in detail the steps that you should follow and the reasoning for each step, so that you are aware of what is happening in the background, and also every stage is essential and the reason it should succeed, so my suggestion for you to note down your notes on an index card, I'll be sharing useful tips, what to look forward to when reading my tale, and also an approach to follow-up with the steps. Now, the process will be explained in those explanations. It will not be a 1-2, 2-3, 4-4 3 4 magical formula because of the reasons I mentioned to you. Keep that in mind.

The information that is compacted and easy to use will be of extremely helpful to you during this process, or in the event that you prefer to highlight the phrases that require action from your side, then at some point when it is time to begin, you could use your notes or resume, or whatever you decide to utilize to begin.

Another reason to take your time reading this before you begin your action is that you need to have a clear idea of what you can anticipate, and what steps you'll have to traverse I would like you to be able to see the bigger picture , similar to studying maps before embarking on your journey. I'll devote an entire chapter to what you can expect, so you are able to set expectations clearly However, I'd like to make a note of a disclaimer that the information I'm going to write about will be based on my experiences and, as it is an individual human body, you can't anticipate the same things that you will experience, even the most factors like age, gender etc. are similar to mine but it is not likely that your body's response will be exactly the same way as my body did. I doubt that both of us will feel anxious similar to me for instance although in the general sense, you'll experience common phases, but with your own unique manner. Let's now get your mind trained and prepare for the next step.

Chapter 2: Beginning Of Changing Your Mind.

From now on, I will delve into the issues of the mind, attitude, etc. through this chapter, to the point where it may seem like I've lost track of the principal subject, but keep in mind that the root of the problem is where we must work on it in order to solve the problem. Since the root of the issue lies in the mind, I will devote certain paragraphs to the general issues of the mind so that you will be able to subconsciously shift your thoughts, feel encouraged and encouraged.

If we're dealing with the mind like we do today it is essential to engage in constant repetition, not basic understanding. You are aware of the most beneficial habits for living a the best and healthiest life However, it doesn't mean you must do them, because with the mind, things become more complicated and simpler in the same way. repeating something at a sufficient amount of times, and you'll create a habit that you will follow and once the pattern is set in your subconscious, you'll keep doing it with no conscious thought on your side, until you develop a new pattern that is at odds with that pattern and changes the pattern.

If you design an pattern and you have no other forces that can alter this pattern, you'll do it forever, that's why you began addicted to smoking the first time and you broke the inertia barrier by repeating the same habit until it was fixed. but with the terrible negative side effect of dealing with a powerful and addictive chemical substance, that acted as a catalyzer in order to make the habit faster and more deep-rooted.

One good idea to instil into your head is to believe that you don't have an issue, don't think of it as a burden, which can only serve to derail your goals, human beings like all other creatures descended from nature is prone to expand and grow and expand, so don't believe you have an opponent to fight, since you'll end up with a sword that is facing your own shadow, consider this as a test and an opportunity to learn which will expose what you're in a position to accomplish when you put your mind about something, once you have mastered this mentalally, you will discover that this is a more comfortable journey that you can undertake, and will reveal to you what are are made of, how powerful you are and that there's nothing in your challenge you won't be able to be able to conquer with enough willpower with focus and determination. keeping an eye on the positive side of everything will provide you with a good starting point for any race, giving you a an advantage that is worth it, and this isn't an exception. always staying ahead of the game.

The way to achieve success is essentially having a clear goal, attempting to fail, then correct the error and try again, continue going, and never give up until you get to the destination you want to reach. The process is no any different. You should be aware of the fact that there are the option to fail, and then get up and continue walking. to date, no one has fallen once in this method, which is an amazing feat that I am extremely happy about, however to be honest, I haven't tried it on such a large scale, as I plan to do following these guidelines, so now comes the real test. I am sure you won't be the firstto fall, however, if you do there are guidelines to follow to get and get back up and continue on your way, and the reason I'm saying this is that I don't want you think that you're a failure in the event of a failure, because no worthwhile accomplishment has been achieved without a single failure. it's a part of the process particularly when there is no rulebook to follow, or instructions or any other kind of instructions. There will be rules in this instance, so I hope that you will not fall one time, but if there is a chance, do not glance at yourself, don't be embarrassed about yourself, simply stand up and walk on with (if you are able to) more determination.

This is the thing that separates winner from loser. Also, think for a second how you'd feel about your life if you didn't be faced with challenges such like this one? Your life wouldn't have any value, at least from a standpoint of growth, and eventually become depression as I mentioned earlier each creature of mother nature has an expanding instinct, which makes it constantly grow and strive for an enriched and meaningful life. This is only possible by overcoming challenges and completing quests and headwinds, the obstacles and traps that throughout these we develop, and planes are able to rise against the wind under the wings. So, this is yet another one of the challenges you'll have to face, and will help you grow stronger, more knowledgeable, and more free to live your life to the highest degree.

In no way should never feel ashamed of yourself, depressed or depressed beyond assistance, which can create an unmotivated attitude before you ever begin. even if you've failed numerous instances before (as I did prior to when I learned this technique) it is not advisable to use this mindset of defeat Failure is only temporary so long as you're determined to get up and go for it.

The self-image that you project about yourself plays an significant role in the success of your life This is true to all the things you've accomplished and are planning to perform in your life. Have you ever been in a situation as a child playing in the park, preparing to jump over a perceived by you, huge ditch that was a real problem for you at that time? Do you remember that feeling of confidence and the fact that you were able to succeed? I'm betting you felt it, and the reverse is also true. in the event that you had a feeling for a few seconds prior to jumping to the point that you weren't going to be able to do it and then jumped anyway, I'm sure you felt a little tense and then you were able to prove you were right. In this case, the famous quote from Henry Ford is applicable "Whether you think you're capable, or you believe you can't, you're correct".

Mentally, too and is crucial and plays a self-image is a key factor in your success The most effective method to achieve anything is to first be sure you're capable of it do it, and then be able to do it. I was unable to play a difficult guitar melody in the past, at least for 15 years. I believed this was not within my capabilities but then I decided to myself "what do I have to do is it, I can! I will not stop practicing until I can play the song with ease, and I am able to impress my own emotions and personal impressions by interpreting it, without sweating and pounding the notes while I play through the song" And guess what occurred? After that shift in my mindset, it took me just several days to get the change real. All the years I believed I could not get out of my own mind, I was actually locked in my own thoughts, the prison was my own that I was causing harm to myself and not even conscious of it. Think about it, I am sure that you've been your own prisoner in many other ways that you have been in, aside from the addiction you're trying to eliminate.

Things that were thought impossible for centuries were made possible when somebody did it and a line of people achieving similar feats took place in only a couple of months. If you need two examples of the first person to conquer Mount Everest as well as the very first who ran a mile in less than four minutes Edmund Hillary with Tenzing Norgay and Sir Roger Bannister respectively, a huge crowd was there to support them in their respective achievements. 1,400 people have completed the mile in under four minutes since then, and 4,000 have reached the summit of Everest in the last few years, since the label "impossible" had been removed the climbers.

The repetition and appear to be off-focus is not a mistake, it's what it is supposed to be. The subconscious mind has control over you regardless of what your conscious mind understands and comprehends. The only way to create an impression on your subconscious is to repeat the same thing over and over again when you have an idea that is deeply engraved on the pattern, your behavior and beliefs will alter for the better, even though you may be aware you are aware that smoking cigarettes is not a good habit does not mean that you are able to give up smoking because you are in control of your emotions which are controlled as a puppet controlled by your subconscious mind, therefore it is obvious that the main reason that we must address exactly there, in the subconscious. And it is the sole way you can achieve it is by repetition and repetition is the only method by which one alters their behavior and develops behaviors of any kind, and when you notice that I describe the identical concepts in different terms do not take my explanations as a joke and think "yes I know this, so what's the next step?" because that won't aid your cause, instead, you should take time to think about and time and again repeating the same approach from the various angles suggested.

When it comes to the mind, it is a known truth that your potential within it is so large that it's much greater than anything any scientist could ever imagine or predict and the decision to stop smoking poses no threat to your mind's actual potential, in fact the capacity of every man who has ever lived is the same to yours. It's an issue of knowing how to harness your mind's subconscious to get whatever result you want, it is one of the strongest tools that you ever use, it's an extremely broad topic that I suggest you study and understand it. Don't lose sight of this concept that the power that your thoughts can bring is unlimited.

In addition to my intention to help you get free of smoking cigarettes or other addictive behaviors I'd be happy to provide a reward to those who share other ideas like those mentioned in the previous paragraphs, as a bonus with the aim of contributing beyond the primary goal and allow you to live an enjoyable life in the broadest sense in the end it is if this can help you stop smoking, but also develop as a person and having an improved understanding of your the habits you have and your general behavior can also improve your overall health. It is important to keep in your mind that we are creatures of habit and they can make or destroy us.

Imagine your the habits you practice as bricks that form your character. The highest quality and best place to be in will result in more positive outcomes for your life. The best method to make a difference in your own life is to select your own personal habits rather than taking them from your educational process without hesitation and blindly following them and never using your personal standards to decide which ones to remove, stress-test, and modify them. If you're stuck in the same pattern of behavior that you were born with, as the majority of us do, then you are relying on practices that were created long before your birth to live in a society that is completely different from the one we live in today. These habits were shaped by a wealth of information today thought to be outdated or incorrect. I hope that this helps you be the best and ignites some part of you to attain new heights that are not tied to our current subject of study Now let's take a leap back.

Don't worry about whether you're mentally prepared to handle this challenge or not, the power that your thoughts can bring is unlimited as you discover more about it, the more you will be amazed at the possibilities even if you're unaware of the possibilities. We live in a world that doesn't support mental growth to reach your potential. However, this does not mean that you aren't capable of it. Now is the ideal opportunity to investigate and discover what you are competent to do, reluctance isn't going to help you improve and will decrease your will power. And determination will play an crucial role in the success that you're about to achieve.

Your brain is superior to the most sophisticated computer technology humans have been able create, and yet , we only utilize a small fraction of our capabilities There are a myriad of books to assist you in understanding and developing your mind. I'm not going to discuss this subject in depth right now, but I am certain you've encountered crossroads which forced you to take crucial decisions, and those choices you made with determination, focus with courage, determination and focus I am sure that if that you did not have one doubt in your head. You'd be able to emerge with a clean slate I'm sure you were able to.

The most important thing to remember is that, as was stated earlier the ability to comprehend is crucial and you must keep at heart that both the strength of your mind, and the drive you need to be successful, are both in your grasp as energy waiting to be unleashed through your determination. You are able to tackle issues that are hundreds of times more challenging than this one this shouldn't be a hindrance to you from pursuing your goals. You should put aside any thoughts that say that you won't succeed because it isn't the case, do not let your thoughts sabotage you by beliefs, you might be a little hesitant in making decisions but not in terms of potential. Keep your eyes on your goal and real magic will emerge.

If you've got the determination, dedication, and an unwavering desire to make the possibility of a breakthrough that will improve your current situation, then you are ready to move on to the next step. I have stressed the subject of mind repeatedly because it is essential to your success in the job at hand, as the majority of errors occur in this field.

Be sure to keep your eyes and guard your thoughts on what you think about yourself and, by no means within the world, allow the notion that you're weak or you are too difficult for you. Get out of these thoughts as soon as they pop into your mind. Don't let your willpower be sucked by any thought or notion of that kind. You could get additional help with this by reading self-help or positive books, speaking to your loved ones or a friend and listening to positive music and so on. for a few good strategies and suggestions.

Be aware that at all times, you're tired of this addiction and will not let anything stand in your way of getting it under control, and making your life better, you could be your most feared foe or best companion, the decision is yours.

At the moment you're thinking whether you should do this on you on your own, with no disclosure to others about what you're doing or whether you can openly disclose your plans and intentions to your family and acquaintances. I'm not sure of a definitive answer to this dilemma I believe it all is based on your personal style and how you feel at ease with dealing with problems. This is your personal decision and if you're married, I think it that at the very least the person you love is aware of what you plan to accomplish, the reason being that you'll go through certain stages where you will not even be able to recognize yourself. I'm not saying that in a positive way. there will be times when you don't recognize yourself and having the support of a partner is essential, one must realize that certain reactions you experience result from internal chemical imbalances that is a natural reaction of your body due to the fact that you're not supplying the substance you are addicted to, and it will be fighting against you to try to replenish the supply and your spouse shouldn't consider your reactions to be an aspect of your normal behaviour and, of course, personal since you may appear aggressive and be easily upset. This is not going to ever be the same, your body will eventually adjust and adapts, however, there is a phase of detox that you must go through and I'll provide further details in the future and also an example of my own.

Chapter 3: What's To Come And The Best Tools To Help You On Your Journey

This section will comprise an amalgamation of my experiences along with the things you need to know and be prepared for, as well as some tips I would advise you take note of and, in the end, I will cut these lines with the determination to tell you the things I would like to hear involved in the process that might help me.

In my experience, I realized that one of the most difficult obstacles to overcome was the one of smoking and drinking both of which are closely related to one another in the case of smoking (if you're reading this article because it is to stop drinking, then you shouldn't be paying attention to this section) The initial thing that I took on when I was a non-smoker the next day was to go to the shop and buying two beers with the goal of mentally dissociating the two activities and, of course, this should not be done in the presence of any abuse, and the goal isn't to replace habits for drinking.

As soon as I began drinking my beer, my mouth began to feel weird it was hard to describe but it was excessively watery. I immediately was prompted to drink "something other" to counterbalance it and then I realized it was a wise choice as I wanted to stay clear the possibility of falling into the most usual trap that I have been caught in by my previous mistakes, which is to go through the week with no smoking, and then completely off track of going out with friends for an alcoholic drink and lighting cigarettes. It is the one of the most common traps to fall into. This is often the result of multiple reasons because alcohol affects the ability of your brain to process information as well as the inner seduction induced by your brain's own desires that is just too strong to resist the desire and you simply slip, so, when you're trying to quit smoking , but you drink and prefer to continue drinking even when it's not a problem for you, you should consider an additional rule to apply for the first four to six weeks when you can only have two drinks when you are out or catching up with a few friends, at the very least until you've completed the detox phase, that is the most difficult for those who want to quit other vices, you should take note of if any of your behaviors are linked to something else, and be sure to remain in a moderate state during this period. If you are a smoker and drinker but are trying to get rid of alcohol and smoking, it might not be the case, but you should to quit smoking cigarettes since it isn't much better.

The process of dissociation went smoothly for me, there was no abuse of alcohol or drinking, and I kept my the amount of alcohol consumed on weekends. The third and second weekends, the task is more challenging I'd highly recommend not to attend any events, parties or any other event which could appeal to you. Your the cravings are at their peak and you'll be at the make it or break it moment when you get this far, it's not an excuse to not do your best, it is a good idea to note down your notes, and note your calendars to only attend events that are it is absolutely necessary to attend an occasion for the family however, if you don't have anything like that Do a favor to yourself and your cause and stay clear of weekends when you go out, particularly those where you'll be in contact with others who have the same addiction problem. but you're in need of a distraction but it's not an issue to sit at your home and observe your hair growing while in front of a mirror. Your hobbies and other activities will come in handy for you, particularly if you're an outdoor enthusiast who enjoys walks or any other kind, then go for it! You can also enjoy gardening, painting or redecorating your home. Keep yourself active and productive, but far from your the mind.

In the beginning days, the dread of the first day is a bit overwhelming You feel strange because you aren't doing something that you're used to doing, and your body begins asking, what's happening and where's my belongings? You're incredibly dedicated and have just begun the new lifestyle, and it's a bit manageable due to this fact, your focus is on the forefront of your mind and you're not easily distracted. However, the difficult challenges are ahead and the fear isn't as strong enough to alter your habits (yet).

What's to come (and pay attention to this) is an increasing anxiety as the days go by. Imagine it as a climb up an uphill slope that gets more and more difficult the your thoughts about "this is too difficult! I'm not going succeed!" will start to get more frequent and become more intense, DISCOVER the thoughts! Your mind and body will begin to nag and punish your body and mind more intensely each day however here's the secret to overcoming all of that. The key is understanding, an enlightened knowledge of what's happening and what you can expect. The main thing you must remember is that this is an infrequent phase that will not last longer than the level of anxiety you are experiencing suggests, and this will only last during the first few weeks, so adopt the attitude of "I knew that this was coming and am aware that it is only temporary" I'd say the first two or four weeks are the most challenging however, once you've gotten past those you will be able to move on from the point. Some addictions might require more time or less time, however the concept is the same. Detoxing your body of things isn't a permanent process, so keep this to your heart at all times, particularly during this phase which is the main way to get over anxiety at times when you need it most.

I realized that the biggest issue with my failed attempts was the assumption that the crushing anxiety would never end and just get worse. But it's not the case. and it gets worse, but it gets to an extent and then it decreases thereafter and this is extremely important to realize, it's just some days, dependent on the specific addiction you have and the circumstances of your body. I'm assuming it won't be an exact amount of time, but looking at these variables I'm not sure it will last more than an additional two weeks to create a total of 3 to four weeks. So that's it! I've given an important piece of advice that is one of the primary strategies to succeed by recognizing that the pain that you'll be experiencing is only temporary and doesn't last for as long as your signs might suggest. The you may feel a craving or desire to get the substance may go beyond that, but you won't experience the overwhelming anxiety, so it's just discipline and awareness to ensure you stay on course and avoid falling for the temptations, which is to say it's not like hunger that comes each and the day This is a different situation it's a detox phase that you must go through It's tough, sure however, it's not impossible especially if you're prepared beforehand and are aware of the things to expect.

Consider this like the equivalent of a race. You know the outcome so you prepare yourself for it. You know that in advance there will be moments when you'll feel exhausted But you also are aware that there is a goal and when you cross the line that is the final destination the same way, when you have crossed your detox point, all that remains will be pure happiness and freedom, as long as you don't go back. for this particular instance, there isn't a precise delineation of where the end line is, but you'll feel more at peace after you have not had any longer a concern, you will feel the urge to eat may be present and absent, but nothing that will cause you to lose control when your resolve is firm enough.

If you believe you'll need psychotherapy for this, don't hesitate and seek it out. Often we need to be able to escape for all the emotions we accumulate in our minds, and those feelings usually are the root cause which causes us to fall into unhealthy habits like those you're trying to break and that is a crucial argument to be made, it's obvious that the issue is in the mind. A good therapy provider will greatly aid the cause. The counselor can assist you in getting your thoughts straight, and offer directions and other guidance to help you get moving in the correct direction. Do not neglect your mental health by pursuing this approach if you feel overwhelmed in confusion, helpless and helpless..

For those who are looking to eliminate another chemical substance, there is one thing I'm going to declare. Certain substances are more powerful or addictive than other, and this can cause the experience to be milder or stronger. I'm not convinced that the time required to detox should alter as much as it has been explained in the past, however the intensity of anxiety may be so intense that it causes hallucinations, sweats, nausea or hallucinations. The symptoms mentioned above are often connected to substances that are likely illegal, so if this is your situation, you should to consult with a doctor in the field of healthcare during the process as it could require additional medication to reduce the anxiety levels, but in the case of alcohol or tobacco this won't be the case and I've detailed my addiction and why I experienced that level of anxiety. It was manageable. Hopefully for you it will be similar.

To help you stay on the right track to get through those tough days during the first week There is an additional tool that might be handy , either a wall or desk calendar. Something you are able to keep your eye at at a close glance regularly, on a daily basis, and usually not your calendar you have on your phone and something that you can keep track of the days that pass by to create an easily visible tool to track your progress. You could set a date in advance for that you are in "goal Phase One" with an estimated time of between two and four weeks from the start date (starting date to be specified later) In this ensures that you always be reminded that this is a temporary phase , and that you are working toward the final goal as time goes by.

Knowing and assessing the progress you're making helps you stay on track. After that, you can move forward two weeks after you have completed "goal stage one" and note the "goal second phase". The first date you mark on the calendar is a reference to the upward period of anxiety (i.e. detoxing) and you'll begin the descent when you've reached that point the second goal phase date will show the progress of a subsequent phase in which you are still feeling anxious but close to being done. The end date can be marked approximately 6 months following the first day that you began, at that point you'll be done. the next time you smoke, it is most likely due to individual choice and not because of an addiction habit.

When you begin, don't just note the milestones you have set, but as the days progress, you can cross them off your calendar, so that you get that feeling of progress . You can also observe the days as ones you've left behind, this will increase your confidence and self-confidence as your move towards your goals. If a child is saving money to buy something, it makes him see all of the money together and believe that he is moving toward his goal Things don't change in this way.

The feeling of improvement in this situation is more emotional and it's crucial to have a reference point that gives you a precise picture of your progress. To keep track of your progress without any references will be difficult since anxiety, while rising at first, it can be as a rollercoaster, with the occasional downs and ups however, the feeling of progressing of it is something that eventually experience through anxiety levels, however, being too focused on things in the moment makes you lose your perspective on the current situation. Therefore, you need to you can influence your mental perception positively by using this simple but effective tool to monitor your progress over the long days and keep your feet planted and focused.

The benefit of this method is that it is much easier to progress with clear vision of the final goal. It is much more difficult to achieve progress when you've got no idea where you stand and also with the awareness that this process is going to be temporary , and the software monitoring the various phases and allowing you to control your thoughts and not let the tricks that your mind to hinder you. using the same metaphor of climbing the mountain, it will be much easier to do it on a bright, clear day where you can always see how far off the summit you are, rather than climb it on a cloudy, rainy day where you aren't sure how long you've got left and whether you're going be able to complete it. It is important to stay focus, and remember that anxiety tends to increase as time passes when instead of feeling that you're progressing, your mind may suggest that you are not, which is the reason failure happens all the time.

What happens to the experiences of the really tough days? The days that will be those ones when your behavior changes as you treat people whom you love terribly without knowing it, you'll be rude to them, or be angry, tiny things will bother you too often, you'll be frustrated with all things, and you will be very negative. This is the reason why I strongly suggest you speak to your spouse, if you are married, as well as other family members living with you. They must be patientand understanding because you're doing this for them. engage in a heart-to-heart chat in advance and inform them that you've read this and they should be aware of about what is expected, but most of all, realize that your emotions are going to be in control, trying to get you to abandon your efforts with every dirty method they can. Depending on your character , this could be a nightmare however, as we have repeatedly said that it is only temporary. two weeks to pay for the cost for a lifetime of freedom is well worth the price.

If you continue to treat people you love dearly and constantly apologize, do so when you feel that you are clear. If this is difficult for you, you can use sticky notes that are attached to chocolates, or other items similar, which can reduce tensions between family members , colleagues at work, and all the general people you share a relationship with or around. I was lucky in this way, as I went through the entire phase, I was by myself, so there weren't any people affected by my moodiness. I do not remember being particularly bad, however I'm sure that I was rude and unruly with a few people.

I can recall vividly the specific incident because it was totally out of normal behaviour, and when it happened , I finally realized what was happening. It was the weekend, and I remember since I can recall that I wasn't looking forward to going to work. I was starving and about to cook breakfast. I wasn't certain what I was craving for, so after mulling about it, I decided for a fry egg, it was a calmed thought moment, which is a proof that anxiety can hit from zero to one hundred in a flash and I decided to turn the oven on and opened the egg gently towards the side of the pan, and as the egg was flowing through the egg shell and into the skillet, I saw that it fell with the yolk breaking, and that was not what I wanted to do When you decide that you'd like to fry your eggs that means you're not planning to make the eggs into scrambled eggs since something went wrong in the unexpected and I took the action that every "normal" person exercising their psychological "sanity" could do: I grabbed the spatula made of metal and threw it on the wall, using enough force that it broke (steel not wood) This is how severe anxiety can strike from the blue.

But what's the most interesting thing? I don't remember being able to explode out of my head. That irrational response was almost automatic and fortunately that's the only insane thing I remember doing in the moment. After I did that, I instantly began to think to myself "What was that? What happened?". It was a brief moment of insaneness and, to be honest, when I started asking this question to myself, I was back to my senses and it was an extreme of stupidity, stress or whatever that was followed by a sanity-inducing moment in which I was able to ask myself about it. Then I realized that it was the detox phase that was playing tricks on my brain and it didn't deter me, but it made me aware of things I was likely to encounter in the near future. I didn't have any guidance in any way as you read this post today, therefore the entire experience was a mystery happening on a daily basis as I traveled I believe that if I had been conscious back then, that you have self-control, I would have found it more rational, straightforward and controlled and controlled. because I'd have been prepared for the unexpected.

and that I would have been 26 years old at the time I'm bringing this information because it allows you to connect to your age as the level of maturity of your brain plays an important role in your personal development. I wouldn't believe that a 45 year old man to be as out of the ordinary as what I've just mentioned, but from an 18 year old man, you could expect similar or more.

Things that are material aren't crucial, they are able to be substituted, but relationships can't and you should be mindful of the way you treat others when you are in your initial phase. keep in mind that any sudden flurry of thoughts in your brain caused by anxiety could turn into a lasting memory of someone you abused and you've heard that those wounds could last for a lifetime. To stay clear of things you could regret, I highly suggest you identify prior to your departure an avenue to release your anger, anxiety and any other blunders you might be guilty of, an exercise program that will really exhaust you such as running, boxing and lifting weights, or something similar to that is a great way to use your favor, and you could supplement it with regular power walks. So make sure you incorporate that into your plan as soon as you get started.

Behavior is controlled by emotions. That's why sudden and drastic changes in behavior can be attributed to hormone changes or brain chemical imbalances eventually, you'll be able to control your own behavior after detox has ended and you'll get more comfortable in your new way of life, this is where your determination to stop plays an vital role. Once you're back in control it's all about discipline to ensure that you don't get off the path, and temptation can seem appealing for a lengthy time, however, it didn't happen to me as I was genuinely exhausted and eager to quit, however I've heard of cases that people don't get rid of the seductive urges be focused in the event that you do In my case, I realized that I fell into that trap when I was in my teens. I experienced a deep swoon and certainly after a few years of being addicted to cigarettes, I was reluctant to put my life at risk which is why I avoided smoking cigarettes, completely aware of the type of situation I might confront if I were to do so. When you've regained your feelings, be careful not to be enticed by the mental traps.

Another thing that could be the case is that you'll feel the strange feeling of wanting something to put inside your mouth, from time every day (this is mostly related to smoking) It is possible to have convenient mints, gum or even candy to satisfy this craving resulting from the habitual smoking however I wouldn't recommend you to fill your body up with sugar. It's not recommended to soothe that feeling by it. It won't assist you, as I'm convinced that it could lead you down an unhealthy lifestyle, and is equally important to recognize and think about, this bizarre desire to put something in your mouth could last for years to become a habit and even after about 16 years I'm still suffering from it even to the present day.

Many people drink coffee, increasing the amount of coffee consumed to multiple cups daily, this does not only have the drawback of sugar, but also the effects of caffeine. If you're a regular coffee drinker, set an acceptable daily limit and also consider that caffeine isn't an invigorating or tranquil substance you'll require, and what I did was adopt the habit of drinking tea without sugar and green tea in particular throughout the day, I would drink up to eight cups per day (that provided me with about 1 1/2 cups in caffeine dosages) however, since it contains caffeine as well and can cause an astringent impact after a few cups (mouth extremely dry) I then mixed it with chamomile tea. The latter is actually a great way to relax and calming, so if you'd prefer to go that route I would suggest balancing with two cups of chamomile tea for green tea. as well as peppermint can be a great ingredient to mix in as it can provide two benefits from this as it helps to reduce anxiety, and something that can assist digestion by taking peppermint. It is known that anxiety and other typical symptoms can develop an acid stomach. Adding caffeine is likely to exacerbate the issue.

You can also conduct an easy search for other plants you can create infusions from, perhaps you suffer from other ailments that can be improved through a specific infusion made from one of the plants to reduce cholesterol levels or other things that could be causing issues for you, specifically, you can kill two birds in one fell swoop.

When it comes to sugar, here are a few helpful tip to help those who are struggling with sugar. Before the tea changes I was drinking large quantities of coffee with the addition of two teaspoons of sugar. then I realized that I was drinking excessive amounts of sugar and it might cause problems for me at some point and, fortunately, before anything regrettable occurred, I made the step of first getting free of all sugar (all it was before I stopped smoking) and I began drinking my coffee without sugar, or any other artificial or natural sweetener. It is important to know the bitterness of my coffee in the beginning. I was used to sweet tastes and it was a sour taste but I stuck to my choice and continue drinking the way I always have, and my consumption of coffee decreased because the flavor did not appeal for me. However, after a few months, my taste began to change and I began to enjoy it. It's simply a matter of getting used to the taste. I've also influenced others at work with the same outcome, but we can't enjoy the taste of sweet coffee. The flavor has is completely different and you appreciate so much more the natural taste of coffee, and you begin to appreciate great coffee for what it really is and if you're looking to eliminate sugar, I highly recommend you follow the same method, and try for a month, without sugar. you'll never regret it I guarantee it.

If you're a work person like me I would suggest you buy a quality travel mug that is insulated to ensure you have an alcoholic beverage for a lengthy time and continue your day by adopting a healthier lifestyle. And if you follow my advice and avoid using sweeteners or sugar and then spill your drink on your keyboard, you'll be grateful, I guarantee it my experiences! It's disgusting to see keyboards covered in sticky residue and, by the way you should get a mug that is spill-proof or one with a top that is well-made to keep your mug safe from accidents. For those who are not in a workplace for most of the time and do an even more active work schedule, I'm not sure which do I suggest, which will depend on the nature of your work as well as your tastes, preferences and the weather, in the case of outdoor activities mostly, but you should be certain to do a thorough analysis before making your decisions and conclusions so that you're prepared ahead of time however, whatever you find appealing to consume, drink or utilize to meet this need avoid eating junk food such as candy, ice cream or other sweets since your weight might increase more than you prefer, which brings our attention to the following subject I'm sure that it is the most typical issue when quitting smoking, so let's discuss the issue.

Weight gain: truth or myth? It is my duty to say that truthfully in both my experience and logic I usually attribute this phenomenon with the following reasons. When you smoke , your body is deeply involved with the task of eliminating harmful substances out of your body so your body has more work to perform to burn the midnight oil each and every minute of the day. The enormous attack of so many chemicals will occupy your system of cleaning like a madman If you quit smoking, you relieve your body from such a difficult task, and your body will be able to unwind and relax, this decreases the energy expenditure that your body used to require previously Another reason could be the fact that people eat more because of anxiety, but those who stopped smoking are eating almost similar foods are also overweight, therefore, I tend to consider the second explanation to be more plausible. more rationally to the phenomenon however, this shouldn't be an issue or anything that is stopping you from doing this Healthy habits can help you to achieving your weight goals as I have stated here. simply work on getting your life to a where you feel happy, relaxed and content as well as..

To combat weight gain and to quit smoking, you can beneficial to follow the earlier suggestion of exercising as an the outlet for anxiety, and all these suggestions contribute to your cause. That's an added benefit of sharing my own experience with the approach I'll be shared in the near future. A good program of cardio that is complemented by more vigorous training can help you build the endurance that cigarettes (or or any addiction) took away from you during the process of cleansing your body's internal organs.

Be aware of this possibility of weight gain. It shouldn't deter you from deciding to go ahead, or cause you pause at all. I cannot stress this enough: being thin to the wrong reasons in the face of the increased risk of heart disease or lung cancer isn't an ideal choice.

Many people consume food due to anxiety, and that's not beneficial for you. If you're a victim of this issue, you should pay attention to this particular phase, because to limit your consumption of tea as recommended, and along with the other facets of no sugar in detail. Now take note of this since it is often missed and is the tiny details that can make the difference between day and night in the end The most important thing to remember for this issue is to ensure that you don't consume more than you feel satisfied. Being satisfied and feeling full are two different things and we are all aware of the difference. If you reach the point that your body saying that no food is required, then you could be suffering from weight issues which is true regardless of a lifestyle like smoking cigarettes or not. A different method to avoid this issue is to make sure you are eating something that is healthy and will benefit your body. For this, you could benefit from smoothies that are mostly made of vegetables. Don't replace it with juices as they are excellent, however, in this instance, one of what we are looking for is the fiber you lack when you drink instead.

The effects of fibers that your body produces makes you feel fuller for longer. It will aid in the metabolization of sugar within your body, creating the perfect cushion against the sugar rush that occurs in the liver. But I'm going to get too technical, and this is just some information I gained along the way and I'm not an expert in this matter , however for your benefit I will pass these suggestions to you. In all likelihood, smoothies made with vegetables are a great way to reap advantages to your body. I cannot suggest them enough, particularly for weight loss.

Relaxing or calming your stress by drinking sugar-free smoothies or teas can assist you However, exercising should be a part of your plan smokers such like I did typically don't exercise. This is nothing shocking about. You'll have a lack of energy to live your day if you smoke so often, so it's not a surprise.

Avoid drinks and processed food while sitting on the sofa watching TV. The majority of processed foods have added sugars and chemicals that can clog the brain and slow down your thinking. They dull your brain and consequently affects your emotional state, which can cause you feeling drained. As stated earlier, emotions determine your actions, and in the end, food can sabotage your efforts and overall well-being It's no way to avoid it and there is no way which will positively affect the cause you are currently fighting for.

Consume a lot of vegetables Your cells require nutrition and, I'm telling you the truth, you'll think more clearly with a healthy diet. The benefits are numerous and this isn't scientific method or an secrets that are not widely known. Everyone is aware of this, which suggests that our behavior is influenced by emotions and not by logic. Most people are aware of what they should do, but their behavior suggests that we do not. Discipline is a must in this procedure Discipline means the capability to issue yourself a directive and then adhere to it regardless of what. You are aware of what you can command yourself since you know what's best for you and it's time to control yourself and establish routines and habits which will improve your life, not take the quality of your life away.

Alongside anxiety and weight management, I'd like to return to the earlier idea of bringing exercise to your daily routine, as it can also improve your immune system. It will help you cleanse your body and mentally, and keep you engaged, motivated with your goals, focused and free, and many more benefits Just consider it this way that your body was created by nature to exercise regularly. in the event that you don't exercise regularly or do it in a way that isn't enough, it will create problems. This logic can be applied to eating healthy, however exercise is the most effective way to combat weight gain, along with the idea of not feeding yourself to the point where you feel content.

Consider the suggestions before starting. Regardless of the you prefer to do for training, develop a strategy to follow. You may want starting small to ensure you don't become frustrated after the third day of pain throughout your body. Make an outline of a specific time to practice on specific times of week. adhere to your plan with a strictness, you could include the and plan to your calendar however whatever your strategy is that doesn't incorporate a the half-hour walk at least three times per week, I would definitely suggest adding those powerwalks in addition to the sport that you like.

Walking is great for your body no matter what your fitness level or age It oxygenates your brain. That's the reason why when you walk, you can think clearly and your circulatory system is optimized and aids in weight management and is uplifting, it lowers the risk of a variety of illnesses, and makes you feel more content and alive. It reconnects you to nature. If you're an observant person, walking could be a perfect time to say your prayers. I'm not able to imagine a better exercise that allows you to think at the highest level while doing it. You come up with innovative solutions to your problems while walking and also you can take it along with your partner to help ease the impact of any mood swings that you might be experiencing, which means indirectly , it can also improve your relationship. The benefits are too numerous to overlook, so add regular walks to your preferred sport to exercise. It's true that I'm repetitive, and I'm attempt to make them seem like a sales pitch, but they're not even part of the process I'll discuss yet, however these tools can boost your odds of success.

In the final aspect of weight control the possibility to turn around is there too, such as a loss of appetite because of anxiety. I've not heard of a person trying to quit smoking smoking and having this issue however, if it occurs to you, it is worthy of mention I'd suggest you consult a physician to find a solution that will bring back your appetite. This is an interim solution.

In any event I have to state that the problem is in the mind like many other issues we have dealt with up to this point, so if you have experienced it and are determined to resolve it from the source and not just the root, something else will be required to manage and direct your thoughts to overcome it. I believe the cause behind this and other mental illnesses is a lack of vision or clear direction (Proverbs 29:18) or, more simply, you don't have a specific purpose in your life that you're working towards If you had one, your mind was designed to stimulate you to find ways to solve issues and guide you on your travels and, of course, the mind that is focused to achieve something worthwhile will not be afflicted by problems that you have to worry you and will not cause psychological disturbances, interruptions or deviations from any kind, because it's completely focused on the goal you have set for yourself.

If you're not able to have an accurate idea of what you're headed in your life, odds are you're dealing with any of these issues which probably led you to an addiction in the first place A mind that is not active can be extremely risky I'm telling you this so that you can engage in an intense discussion with yourself, which could help you to think more clearly and allow you to draw some worthwhile conclusions from the process, but as we're not trying to address the issues here, I'll give you the concepts in a way that will give you.

Another powerful tool to include in your arsenal is meditation. I've seen extremely successful people attribute the success they have had to their meditation and you don't need to be an expert to do it If you are able to get to a state of peace or inner peace, peace and tranquility and sense your self-worth and your potential, then you're well on your way and there's no need to employ an spiritual guide to help through the process. whatever method of meditation you choose to employ is fine sitting down and relaxing and gradually connect with your thoughts, you can accomplish your goals that are a breeze and flow naturally like praying as it is an inner job that is meditation. It's exactly the same (in my personal opinion) it's an internal task If you've never tried it, I would suggest that you give it a go.

There are a variety of meditations you can investigate if you wish to delve deeper into the subject. Study and practice, the most basic I've heard or read about is called transcendental meditation. It's done twice per day, when you do there is nothing to do and nobody can disrupt your practice with a mantra. choose a quiet place and don't lie down, simply sit and take 15 to 20 minutes of practice each time, the concept behind this is to help calm your mind.

The technique I employ was learned in the text "Psycho-cybernetics" from Professor. Maxell Maltz, in his excellent book, he explained how he imagined a location in his head that he visited. I was enthralled by the concept and decided to adopt it for myself. I came up with within my mind a gorgeous Victorian style home that has stunning chandeliers and a piano in the ballroom. The home is situated at the heart of the woodlands next to a lake which only exists in my mind and I return to it whenever I feel like it.

The time you spend in meditation is the most effective way I have found to bring your feelings into alignment with your thoughts. when you can match your emotions with your thoughts, the most significant advantage you'll gain is that this alignment will direct your thoughts to exactly the way you would like them to following your thoughts and conscious thought processes, and because you are controlled by your emotions, that implies that your "automatic control system" will be in control without conscious effort on your part , guiding you to the place you would like to take you. This is something that should be carried out frequently because the reason for this is that we are greatly affected by the environment around us and the results that you have created for yourself may be gradually diverted from your desired direction The process is so subtle that you do not actually notice the changes until you're completely wrong.

Meditation can bring peace to your life It's like cleansing your mind. It can help you get answers to you "out out of thin air" or even when you are doing it for a specific reason I cannot recommend it enough for other aspects of your life, more than just for achieving the aim that brought us here this moment, so this is a benefit.

All of the things listed (healthy eating, exercising as well as meditation.) might seem like a lot to include completely to your daily routine however, giving these things an opportunity in this phase of detox, it will spend a few weeks into them, and it will be extremely helpful as those weeks are the most crucial of the entire process.

Let's now talk about the positive aspects of what you can anticipate, these can be the most relevant to tobaccobecause those are the things I can discuss and relate to however I am certain that if you set out to achieve another objective, your personal habits will show in proper time the advantages of its own when it is gone from your body, which will depend on the goal you are working on. Just think of this as an adventure to see the positive results you'll experience, this adventure can be exciting on the positive aspect too. The reason I put a lot of an effort to highlight the bad part of the story is to inform that you are aware of that you should be prepared, and not as there aren't any nice things to anticipate.

If you smoke a lot, it is most likely your teeth show the appearance of a yellow hue that is noticeable above your natural shade, this is among most noticeable things that I observed. my teeth were whiter, the shade I'm talking about is not a superficial thing, is something that's internal to me as I am not a physician however you can observe it yourself, and it appears like nicotine along with the shade it gives to your body will disappear completely, and this is distinct from the brown stains that you see on the exterior or inside of your mouth when you view at them with a mirror, these are superficial and require professional cleaning. The natural hue of your teeth is affected by your race, do not expect them to be more brilliant than the moon, but a change in color is evident within the first 3 days or at least.

With this change in tone from your teeth at the same time, another aspect you'll observe is your skin. there's something distinct about it. I'm not sure how to describe it. I'm unable to tell if this is glowing or what can it be, but it appears younger, healthier and more natural. It also looks more vibrant, and when I claim that your body is cleaning within is not a joke! This is true! It's probably just water.

The most obvious improvement of course , is energy, you're not out of breath while climbing an uphill slope, or when you run and exercise generally it is a major positive. This alone is enough to justify the effort of quitting smoking, as it can enhances your daily life. Consider this: what could you do with 20% of energy? You could accomplish a lot more.

Another advantage you'll enjoy and perhaps the most obvious benefit is that you don't smell good, and when smoking, you'll be carrying a an unpleasant odor and this is not a secret. It is also true for bad breath caused by drinking and drinking. I'll illustrate this with a tale of my own experience. I recall a time when at the college I was in an 8:30 am class. typically, I smoked before the class began, and this was my first day of classes and the student who was next to me in the class told me that I smelled terrible I had no idea the man, but I didn't mind the rude remarks and went in the class. which coincidentally, the day I quit smoking was shortly after the incident, and I can remember attending a different 8:00 am class, probably one year later, and to my surprise, I was seated next to a fellow student who had has just taken a puff before class began, his smell was so strong it irritated me and it was a shock to my memory of the incident that occurred one year earlier and I realized, "my god! I now understand the remarks I received one year ago. That one was absolutely right! It's awful!" That smell lasted all of an hour and I'm sure it was unpleasant in any way. When you're smelling this way, you don't usually consider it however you can make people uncomfortable, they don't even tell you that it is affecting your social life. Bad breath caused by alcohol can do the exact same effect and so having the negative impact on your life is one of the many benefits that you gain when you reach the end of the road and quit these habits it is worthwhile to mention that I've realized that those who have quit smoking are more sensitive to the scent of cigarettes as people who have never even smoked which was a good thing to me as I was able to stay away from it completely.

Your senses will awaken as your taste and smell senses will be sharpened, and you'll find that what you thought was normal and precise perception of things was actually a numbing of your senses and a common problem with disorders related to toxic substances can affect your senses. Food can taste different, and even the smallest things that happen in your daily things like the scent of wet soil on the rain are more intense. This was a wonderful and exciting discovery for me. You begin to appreciate small things of the world around you.

Cash in your pocket or any other illegal habit comes with a significant tax from governments as well as when it comes to illicit substances, the prices are definitely expensive and the motive behind this tax is quite simple. these substances pose a threat in the health system of any nation, in the event that you consume alcohol or smoke and get ill, the government has to be able to treat in the future, you'll cost lots of money for Social Security and a reasonable solution to the problem is to tax the substances to bring in enough money to tackle the issue it is a matter of mathematics and commonsense.

That brings us to the conclusion that you spend too much on what you consume compared to the expense of making it, yet you pay less when compared to the amount needed to restore your health if you suffer from it. However, this shouldn't be an excuse to be celebrated like you're taking advantage of something. After all, what comfort should you have if the government is there to help you when your quality of life was ruined.

You'll not spend the money that you used to spend. If you look at this amount as a regular expenditure, it isn't likely to impress you however, when you look ahead to the future, you'll realize it's an enormous amount of cash, I can remember when I was in the 8th month after I left, I calculated of the savings and purchased a great watch, which I wear today. There was no reason to keep receiving prizes for overtime since after eight months, you'll know that you're over it and when I conduct calculations today based on the price of cigarettes today and a look at inflation adjusted prices that I can buy an apartment with the money (with considering the economy of my nation and the region) Imagine having a rent-free time compared to having an addiction that takes away the time of your life each day. And a home could be something you be able to pass on to future generations. That's why you'll have additional money to spend.

If you're suffering from frequent headaches, I have great news for you. it's the next benefit to add to the list. Headaches are less frequent (if there is any). One of the primary signs of dehydration is headaches, as well as one of the primary results of smoking cigarettes is dehydration. So it's not a surprise that this benefit exists as you'll be more hydrated even without smoking and it's the same for any chemical toxin. all of them have this in common. They cause dehydration. One way to determine this to determine if you are dehydrated is to check the color of your eyes. Your eyes will appear more vibrant and clear.

I have a friend who used to use a powerful migraine medication Her condition was so severe that natural light could cause headaches. So she had to sleep in a dark room with the blinds closed however, after quitting smoking the migraine completely disappeared without medication. I'm not saying to claim that migraine is only caused by a dangerous substance that is present in our body, since I'm not a doctor and I'm not certain whether you suffer from migraine and whether also be a case for you however it is an opportunity.

Imagine for a moment that you're not just cleansing your body of the toxic substances you're addicted to as well as releasing your liver from the usual task of dealing with other things that are connected to the addiction such as the negative side effects from medication you are taking, this can come from small chemicals like painkillers to medications to lower blood pressure, when it's the result of smoking cigarettes or other harmful behaviors. You might believe that these ailments are more genetics. If you believe this way , take into consideration that just because you're prone to developing them due to your genes does not mean that you're destined to suffer from a condition however, it is certain that your lifestyle could increase the likelihood that you develop health issues. It is also true that there are certain habits that can be used to reverse the effects of bad habits and bring back health. One such habit with which I have come across is the practice of veganism for diabetes type 2 if you are suffering from this disease or know someone who does I would suggest you look into the topic.

Alongside headaches, everything that you could attribute to a an unhealthy circulatory system could be possible benefits when you quit smoking nicotine within your body. The benefits listed so far are the most noticeable, however that doesn't mean that there's not more on the list. Actually, in the benefits list,, the majority of the time you won't notice these, however they will be present, the list starts from the moment you the time you quit smoking, and continue for years when the detox process has reached its maximum. Once you quit smoking cigarettes, gradually the levels of chemical start to drop, and the levels of oxygen within your bloodstream will normalize and the list continues as your cells begin to oxide less and everything in your body. Your body will function better eliminating free radicals, and the list continues.

The healing process will take years. You will notice improvement after a couple of weeks, but the job of your body to keep moving forward although you may not be able to feel any change, can take years. The chances of having a stroke, for example will diminish gradually over time until you are able to have similar chances as smokers who have never smoked I believe I've recently got to that point with more than 15 years.

I'm not convinced that the current research has revealed and revealed the entire negative effects of toxic habits fully, or the undiscovered advantages to eliminating them. do not believe that current research is the only way to know, especially the small portion available to you is everything there's to.

Read testimonials, conduct your own discoveries, look at images of cancerous lungs as compared to normal ones or livers if drinking alcohol, you must awake and look at things as they are. the consequences you'll be exposed to must be well-known to you to assist you on both sides so that you can make an informed decision and also to motivate you to continue your journey in knowing what may be coming to you.

The main point is your body will experience changes, and your mind will change and removing the habit that is harmful is an amazing breakthrough that can bring an entirely new you with benefits that will cause you to think over-the-million dollar issue that has been circling my head for years. Why didn't I do this action before?

Keep in mind that the unwelcome results of the process are only temporary and the beneficial ones will last for a long time Keep this in mind when you begin to notice these effects, this simple fact will boost your enthusiasm by putting things into the right perspective, knowing that you will gain for the rest of your life and what negative side effects will disappear.

Chapter 4: Determination

It will be apparent why it was said to not start after you have read the entire book. You will feel that you are more aware of the implications, and tips and techniques to use that are extremely valuable in the course you'll soon be confronted with, this knowledge can greatly increase your odds of success. I also gave you a set of tools to assist you in fighting as we to be able to tell the best way to proceed in the event that you decide to adopt the same route I took to get rid of my addiction But first, I would like to thank you for taking the time for getting to this point as it indicates that you have given a seriously thought to making changes to your life for the better, and I believe that I've influenced you to not just change your lifestyle, but to more positive changes, too like the other ones in this book have done so far.

Similar to the way I've described so far, the modification of the system requires you to think from your part to adjust the process to your particular actual situation, requirements such as. In the next section, I will present the principles to be followed and then you'll think and calculate to ensure that the rules are applicable to you. This is due to the fact that each of us is unique and are faced with different challenges so it's not the same magic formula that could apply to an 18-year-old young man that it would be to a 40-year-old one. Also, a low-income person doesn't have the same set of rules to consider, as will one with enough wealth since (spoiler warning) the money factor will play part of the equation (and you don't have to worry you won't have to worry about the money to me, but don't believe you've found the answer since there's none and you'll be able to be able to see the difference as we get there).

Let's now jump into the business. The first thing you'll need to take is be 100% sure that you're in this and that there is no way back, and that you will destroy your bridges while you're on the road This determination is the defining factor of your process. Without it, there is a chance of failure make this decision like your life is on the line and, to some extent you will know that it is.

If you have to wait a couple of days to reflect before making a decision make it happen, there are various levels of conviction and we want you to have the highest level and write down the reasons you'll take the plunge regardless of whether you choose to do so, since during times of stress, they'll provide a solid reminder of why you are doing this when you feel anxious and your mind starts playing tricks on your mind. Your determination is the foundation of your process, so don't make this task lightly.

Make a list of everything, regardless of whether it's your children or your family as well as your health, determination to live, the improvement in living quality to protect a relationship, everything should be documented. Also, if you could make a list of your list in a laminated form and keep it around in your purse, that will be the next device to help you manage your system. Every when you are feeling anxious or feel vulnerable and weak make a list and increase your motivation to persevere. Sticky notes are best kept on your computer's display If you are spending a lot of time in there, or on your nightstand, it may appear odd, but you'll only have to look at them during the first few weeks, which are the more complicated ones.

It's time to consider if the relationship prompted you to begin and then isn't working out, or goes off the rails or ends in a break-up during the course of your journey, if that's the case don't stop there Continue I'm certain there are plenty of other motives to keep going, and it's unlogical to ascribe motives to someone else from yourself. A relationship is an effective motive, and it's true, but don't be a slave to something that's not entirely in your control to dictate the direction of your life. the weak times should not be used to excuse a slide, because your mind is extremely powerful and only you have charge of it. External factors will only have an impact if they are allowed to make an impact on you "An entire ocean of water will not sink a vessel unless it is able to get inside the vessel" Goi Nasu.

So, head to an area that is quiet and don't allow anyone or anything to disturb you. Go to the countryside and sit among the trees, visit an empty church or a location which you're not familiar with such as a room in your home. Don't bring your phone along It's the intention to get you out of your everyday routine and gain fresh eyes and begin your own thinking. You should give yourself plenty of compelling reasons and don't forget to record your thoughts down.

Don't consider whether you are able to do this or not, it is not relevant at this point and you need to make an emotional leap over at this point, letting go the influences of your previous experiences, beliefs, and especially don't let yourself be influenced by previous failures (if they have already occurred) and you should make this choice with the conviction that whatever decision you make is going to prevail, and you're in total influence over its outcome. let me apply an analogy to help clarify this idea You should make your decision like you're standing at a show in a shop, looking at the item you're contemplating buying, consider that you have the cash than you will require to complete the purchase, i.e. money will not be the primary factor in determining whether you'll purchase the item or not. It's only a matter of decide whether you want to buy it or not and nothing else matters as a millionaire contemplating purchasing a candy bar , so of thing that he doesn't need to look at the cost that the chocolate bar comes with as there is no doubt that money won't be a barrier in the way if you decide to purchase the item. In reality, this analogy isn't as far off from the truth. like I said that you've got infinite possibilities stored in your mind and your brain will carry out the work, and you're a millionaire and if you've experienced previous mistakes, you can look at these like if the millionaire (yourself) was at the same event, and forgot to carry his wallet at the time, but this time the book will become your wallet, therefore, you won't have to think about it because you've got the ability in you.

It is essential to consider from that point forward, actions that are inspired. Action and inspired action is two different completely different things This distinction may not be apparent from the perspective of a third party but all you see is the person doing any act that is viewed as simply motion, however in the world of the invisibly is more rich than the action that is inspired, it is the most significant thing in the world, especially if you've noticed that the universe opens windows or doors when other doors close due to this There are many books that deal with this issue and are not the subject of our discussion this moment, however the coincidence of things aligning when you are determined is a fact and is only one part of it. Also, it alters your character just like steel once it is tempered. it's very difficult to fall down if you take this approach while if you do something based on inertia alone, the slightest interruption could alter the course of your action and create doubts over whether you're going in the right direction.

Inspiring action is a powerful force with a lot of energy attached to it and that force, though not seen is able to generate enough leverage by the will to act as if it were fuel. This combination acts as an exploding ball, destroying any obstacle or circumstance that hinders achievement with grace and grace that is effortless. That is why I am determined in this point. When you have reached this level of belief, you're almost to achieving your goal.

If a couple of weeks isn't enough, you can take the time you require to, this is the most crucial step to accomplish these kinds of goals, it's the base of the system we'll construct, and you'll be able to tell what happens when you build on poor bases (Matthew 7:24-27). It is important to have this process in place as only a single shot, in the beginning I pointed the fact that this is mostly an internal process that requires your mind repeating the same thing repeatedly is necessary to impress your mind which is why I seem to sound like an old record a lot of times and I apologize for that, however there is some reason for that. I've always believed there is a point of the mind at which you are able to see everything clearly regardless of what topic you're talking about It's a place that everything is black or white. You might be confused by something , but once some sort of reasoning occurs, or you locate the answer to your question in an article, or talk to a person or after a few minutes, things begin to settle in your head and appear clearer, and you get to the point where everything is either black or white. The gray scale fades when you're there, and answers become to be as clear as pure crystal. There's no hurry when you are stuck somewhere on the gray area in your thoughts and aren't sure how to proceed, i.e. whether you're ready stop for good and stay for the rest of your life or not, you should look deeper into your brain to discover a clear solution to your question. The most important thing to remember is don't try to force things, and don't make decisions just because you believe you need to. The idea is to that you do things because you desire them from your heart, that's what we want to achieve.

Engage your mind until the desired level is attained. There are pros and cons for the majority of decisions that you'll encounter in your daily life, and for a successful implementation you must be completely certain that you are in the right direction, and I am certain you already know this. When you're in line with either the black or white and every action you take to go in the right direction in your mind screams that you are getting there, and when you are moving to the opposite direction,, you are able to feel it immediately Your internal guide system is alerted immediately and I cannot overstate this enough: it is imperative to burn your bridges and not be able to go back after you've reached the point you will be able to burn them.

Chapter 5: Consciousness And Unconscious Alignment

In a non-threatening or in survival mode the subconscious mind operates automatically in short-term satisfaction, unless it receives received a different message from the conscious brain. The short-term reward isn't an any exception which is why you were hooked to begin with regardless of whether you begin to experience satisfaction from being accepted by the same group of addicted individuals you wanted to connect with or the dopamine surge result of the substance that is toxic that you are addicted to, in the end it is irrelevant and we're on the process of getting out of the rut, but it is crucial to understand this concept, as the next step is to provide your subconscious mind with the new direction of getting rid of it.

Remember that you are governed by your emotions that are stored in your subconscious. So it is time to "educate" it. We must demonstrate to it what you're looking for so that it will support your efforts rather than thwarting them. This may seem light or unimportant however it is extremely important and I attribute to this idea the effectiveness of this method, due to the determination was the only thing I needed to do at instances where I failed however the one shot I took to this method that I tried during the process, was the one that I could get my self out of the hole that I was in. So, don't ignore this idea that you have to alter your subconscious's thinking to get to the destination you want to reach. If you can grasp this idea well, it applies to all areas of your life, and this is yet another golden point for you to have stayed with me to this point.

Concerning the programming If you've achieved the necessary degree of commitment the next step we must take is to eradicate the psychological roots in the addiction from the brain that is where the habit's roots are. If you were to suffer today from amnesia and you were to relapse, would you have the habit? Do you think you are continuing to be "in in love" with the person that you have an unhealthy relationship with? Most likely, not. If you're wondering why I speak so often about mindset in my book relating to quitting smoking or other vices, this is the reason.

This will require time and effort This step of the process will be similar the process of putting bricks, one at a time to be erected until the wall has raised, think of an equilibrium scale, with an enormous burden on the other side . you gradually place a burden onto your side until the needle moves slowly till the needle of balance is pointed toward your side, which is precisely what this will be.

Gradually, but gradually, your old habits will gradually become less effective and the new one (or lack of) will grow stronger in small increments. Behaviors can be created this way. How many times did your mother insist that you brush your teeth before you got used to it? What would happen If she had only asked you one or twice during your entire growing up years?

It will take some time as the subconscious mind must be enthralled the concept. It is not simply a matter of grasping, but more a issue to "hit on the right nail" until the nail is fully put in place.

If you do not make this programing the goal, any attempt to get rid of addiction, or any other habitual behaviour that is superglued has slim to no chances of success since eventually, the force of the program will pull you into a vicious force that you are unable to combat.

Did you notice that there has been no time until this point have I been requesting you to avoid smoking a cigarette? It's not an accident, nor I'm going to begin yet (it is likely to happen in the near future) However, now, what I'm going to request is that each moment you light a cigarette, in the event that you decide to, you must think with all your heart that your smoking days have really over and that you are taking a break from it. This change in consciousness and feelings is actually the beginning of the programming process we just mentioned and prepare you for the next stage that are to come. Feel that you're in control and that this is the final chapter of your time as smoker (or drinker, or whatever it happens to be) It will feel similar to telling your body "enjoy the moment because it's going to last long" like that You can feel the power and the determination increase inside you as you repeat these words over and over again. Feel how your determination and strength increase each day over the next three weeks or so that is the time for the programming section, which is extremely crucial. If you do as this article outlines, it will place you in control. Take these lines and read them repeatedly until you can make them well, as If you've attempted with determination before giving up and did not succeed, you're missing the piece accountable for your failures.

It will be a time period not more than 3 weeks, unless exceptional circumstances. Consider 3 weeks if:

* You're still healthy i.e. you're not reading as you've already been diagnosed with something that makes you want to give up.

* There is no illegal more potent toxic habit that requires a higher level of focus.

Your work, or family relationship isn't just a thin layer of ice close to breaking and you are confident that you can be patient and program your brain.

If you believe you can do that in three weeks in a breeze and give 3 weeks' notice period to your subconscious mind for programming and you're able to proceed.

If you're already convinced to go on and think that you don't require 3 weeks, you could cut one weekoff, but less than two I'm not sure it will assist much as it is essential to begin laying an emotional foundation for your new routine (of absence of the previous unwanted one) prior to the date.

I'm not saying that I'm not encouraging you to continue intoxicating yourself for over the next three weeks, but you might want to make use of this time to reduce half the dosages, or even stopping smoking altogether or reduce the amount in increments of the amount you feel at ease with, but think of the next 3 weeks as an "test run" and, if you don't succeed during this test take your time and don't be overly much since you haven't yet reached day zero yet, or the start of the initial phase on your calendar. I have been guilty of enjoying the 3 weeks I had back then I didn't stop any of my cigarettes (not telling you to do it also, but that was my experience) I remember the mantra I repeated to myself over and over and again each when I smoked that these were the final days, and they were.

Remember that we mentioned earlier that your mind is an ocean vessel that turns the steering wheel. It will take some time to begin moving in the direction of the new direction and feel the effects of the turn, not like a car which at the same time when you start turning the wheel, the car instantly turns? From now on, you'll be making the steering wheel turn in your mind. This is the reason we're giving you this time frame to adapt internally and this time be able to control your thoughts gradually, putting tons of weight on the scale for your benefit It's just a matter of time, that's how it operates.

This is again the result of a mental process and feeling. It is now time to get your subconscious mind to believe that by that it is telling you with every idea of where you're headed to from now on It should be aware that the next era is on the way and it needs to be in tune with the coming days with the new lifestyle you'll soon be living.

The idea is to shift your thoughts throughout the day that whatever you're doing, whether it's smoking or whatever else happens to be in the near future, will come close to an end. It's true that this helps greatly, as it allows the time to reflect internally to prepare your body for what's going to happen. Anyone who prepares for a contest goes through this, regardless of whether it was conducted with conscious thought or not.

A sudden change in direction isn't something your subconscious mind is designed to accomplish, so having a predetermined date for when it should begin, will also train it to do so to be able to align the directions you wrote upon it with the result of directing you by your senses to get to wherever you'd like to take you. Certain plastics break easily when you attempt to bend them using pressure, however, when you heat them gradually and in a gradual manner, but not burning them, they'll attain a temperature at which the material is able to do whatever you like using it. You can alter the shape of it to your liking The mind works similarly in that it is slowly and gradually you will be able to master keys.

You need to set this date ahead of time and this is the perfect time to define it. Take the calendar we talked about earlier and mark the date, keep in mind two or three weeks from the time you're reading the following lines. You can read even earlier should you not meet according to the specified criteria.

Another method to influence your subconscious to have the occurrence of a significant event that happens in our lives and will change our current reality. If you've been identified with an event that can't be put off or has an intense sense of urgency it is best to skip this stage, as that the experience of that moment in your subconscious performed the task, and in the event that it didn't, since you'll not have the frame of mind which is among the most vital components of the brain, you need to be more careful when you begin the next step, and establish your own standards to strengthen your customized system and less susceptible to mistakes.

If you've written the day zero on your calendar, it's up to you what you plan to accomplish from now up to that point in relation to your addiction as long as you always have the date set in your mind and realize that it's the final day and keep repeating it to yourself repeatedly. After I mentioned those words to myself, a strange sensation came over me. It's odd feeling that I am sure you will soon will experience it. Your stomach is uncomfortable and you feel anxious and uncertain, but also happy while at the same time. when you begin experiencing these feelings, you're on the right path.

The deadline date or zero date should be the main throughout the day regardless of whether you smoke or not. I have lived as if that was the case, especially when I lit my last cigarette, the that you have read about. the thought kept going through my mind throughout the day when I lived through those months. Relax on those days mentally.

If you've been in a state of denial because of addiction, think like you're watching the prison window and enjoy the day outside, knowing that you'll soon be freed from the prison. Anything that helps you to overcome the mental hurdle will help.

Chapter 6: Day Zero

When the day is over is the real challenge So far, you've done your best, but it's only your mind and your subconscious will be already trained and aware of the new direction you're going, therefore it will cooperate with you. You may feel a craving, but your inner self are likely to feel something is off when you do get caught up in them, this is your subconscious working for rather than against you. You've been prepared for the challenges that will occur during this phase. This is the day that you'll actually be clean and the detox process will begin (if you've not actually stopped your addiction during the training run) However, we must to be sure that you don't slip and that someone is watching you.

It is true that no one is able to watch you 24/7 except you, and you're the one person in this endeavor. attained, therefore you'll be your own personal policeman, or constantly watching your camera recording your actions. You can be a secretive person to me, or any of your family members or friends however, you cannot conceal from yourself. And the promise you made for this particular system is only with you, and you agreed to each side of your agreement Let's now be sure that it's legally binding.

My personal experience with the pledge was made with acquaintances, but eventually within my circle it was made publically, so everyone knew the difference. The fact that people began to see me sans a cigarettes (or the smell of one) was quite noticeable as well as some of my friends who weren't part of the group were able to offer me a drink while drinking a drink with them the opportunity to smoke a cigarette, but they promised to keep it private at the time of week 2. I never felt like I was being tempted, it was obvious to me that the real dedication was not to those that were not present and myself, but rather with myself. it was a personal thing for me so I resisted any similar offers.

Your situation should not be any different. We are trying to make your life better, not to find ways to fool ourselves, there's no way back. If you begin to feel that things are becoming extremely difficult, you need to seek help, but do not cheat, and never forget that it's a mental problem, so if you require assistance, seek it out the way you need it and in your head in the event that you are suffering from one of those extreme instances of secondary reactions which require an appointment with a doctor however, do not take medications that do exactly the same thing into your body. e.g. nicotine patches for those who smoke. you're not searching for alternatives, and we've made it obvious prior to.

The motivation for your mind may be derived from heart-to-heart conversations with the people you value in your life who can keep you motivated If you've recently began to exercise, setting objectives related to it can be extremely beneficial and will direct your attention to a particular goal and you will not lose focus on your desired objective, which could be to walking up to 5 miles in each week's increments, if you have began by doing a "walking therapy" like the one we discussed earlier and enhance its results through listening to music that is positive or inspiring podcasts..

Once you reach this point, after you've been working internally and you feel powerful there are hints of doubt within your mind but they aren't too loud, you'll feel confident that you have made a deal, and there will not be any turning back. This will take some period of time and you need to ensure that you get maximum benefit from your enthusiasm.

The key to inspiration is at this point, think about you throw a few nails in a desk and they start all over the place with an unorganized final view. What happens when you are close enough to an incredibly strong magnet? It will align all of them in the same direction and restore harmony and order. This magic effect can be replicated exactly the same way after your mind is in sync with creativity. Your thoughts, feelings, goals and actions will be aligned just like the nails are to the magnet. The more motivated your life is, the lesser self-control you'll need, and the greater your chance of success.

However, no system is perfect without fail protocols to follow in the event that emergencies arise. For instance, if you get off track The possibility of falling down could be minimal by now however, it is not zero and in this case, we must collaborate to create an entirely customized section, to date no one who reached this point using these procedures has fallen and I from the bottom of my soul, I would like to be the first to experience this however, in the unlikely event that it occurs, we must get you back on track, remember that you crossed the day-zero line and now there must be consequences. This isn't a exercise run any more. This is where the financial part comes into play as it is the most modern way of keeping things under control , and we will employ this method to help you get back on track.

Have you noticed it's extremely difficult for someone to can cross a red light in traffic that has cameras on it? If you don't have a real emergency situation or a dead one, or you cross it in a haphazard manner, you'll remain there until the green lights allow you to cross even if it's 2 am in the morning, and there's no one else in the vicinity. In addition to the fact that we're well educated and have a stable society, the enigma of this phenomenon of people crossing the road is, of course, the cost which nobody wants to pay for, and the cameras at the traffic light makes it pretty certain that you'll be fined for crossing if you do compare it to a traffic light which doesn't have one.

You read that right in the event of a fall you'll pay. This is the reason no one has yet fallen because the fine isn't affordable, and when you've got penalties that are far too much, you will give up to good conduct because you are aware of how much it's going to cost you and, now that I've revealed this crucial ingredient of our magic formula, I'll conclude my tale.

My friend and I were at a cafe, and we were discussing about how we had had enough of smoking. Eventually, we came up with the idea "let's put our money on the line!" a bet on which people who smoke would payfor, it was too terrifying to begin immediately, so we decided to give us a couple of weeks to begin to calm our anxieties We didn't realize that we were in the early programming days. However, back then we didn't realize that this was going to be the main element of our success. If someone fails the bet, the person who failed must pay the amount, similar to a swearing jar type of arrangement and then a unanimous agreement was reached and the necessity of defining the amount that was to be paid, after which we came to an agreement on a figure, but we were nervous because it was a lot! and we were worried about paying a large sum of money , both for the amount of money to be paid and also for possible failures that might occur and we were faced with the challenge of deciding what we should do with the money that will surely be collected. It's not an issue because "I fold" this is my money. I'm out. There's no way! It would be too simple to do. This was the kind of per-occurrence deal, much like the traffic light. You go over a certain line, you payand you go back and of course, you pay the same amount, so we thought that a large amount of money would be collected after the three months that comprised three months "bet" (mark the date of your three months following the day you reached zero on your diary). Simple concept, whether you smoke a cigarette, or smoke a cigarette, or whatever and are penalized.

As a large amount of money will be taken (or it was our assumption) we had to come up with a strategy to manage that money, and we spent an hour debating and fighting over the issue. Should we transfer all the cash to two other? No, that's unfair. We came up to the ideal solution, no one can keep the funds, they will be given to charities and we'll decide later which charity. It was the best solution since the agreement created two obligation with one moral cause in case you fail, and the second one for yourself. However, as you know we were pleasantly surprised to discover that three months later, no one fine was imposed and we had successfully quit smoking , or at least at the end of three months for all of us and for the rest of my life.

I'm not able to tell you what amount we were fined without impacting your thoughts thereby the circumstances we faced aren't identical or similar, however I'll provide some information that will help you determine what's the most appropriate sum for your needs. In the past, it was about one third of my monthly income in the year before taxes which meant that I required more than a week of income just to light cigarettes, even a light ones. I've already informed you that it was high as I think the high percentage of success to this fact and the punishment should be so severe that you be thinking twice before committing to it. This is the essence of the system. Don't make it too easy on yourself, think about your current situation as well as the amount you earn and the amount you earn. If you're wealthy and have enough money to solve the problem you can pay for it, then penalize yourself for the hours you spend in community work but not a lot! Similar to what you would do if financially dependent or poor of others. No matter what, you should be able to pay for more than three penalties per month, either in terms of hours or money I'll repeat it again. Don't make it easy for yourself. You'll have to succeed and we'll make it as it is meant to be.

If you don't succeed and have to pay the bill, I'll suggest you to do the same thing that we did back then that you donate to charity, select the charity you feel most strongly with, and that will result in a donation and at the very least, some feeling of comfort in the event that you do fail once or twice however, I can assure you that the framework we've built up for a while is enough to stop you from falling. slip. For a reminder of what to expect, bear in mind the most difficult days are just one or two, and once you've passed those tough days, which , I'd say, are about 2 or three weeks, you won't need to be worried about it. You won't be in a rush or stressed for a long time and there's a conclusion to that, and after these weeks, everything will be going to be downhill after that point.

Make a note of the days on your calendar, motivate yourself by setting a objective in your sport and the stress and internal noise will be reduced to a minimum. I doubt you'll ever have to spend money since I believe you'll be able to do it the way I did and other people have done it, and it's not that difficult when you have a solid, solid method in place, and you now already have one.

Chapter 7: Illusion Of Smoking Cigarettes

Smoking can help you relax.

Many smokers believe that smoking cigarettes aids in easing. However, the truth is that nicotine is a relaxing agent for the body. If you are taking your pulse, then smoke two cigarettes in a row the rate of your pulse will rise significantly.

For many smokers, the most enjoyable smokes is one following eating. The time to stop working is when you have sat down for eating a meal is over. It's a time of relaxation to ease our thirst and hunger. However, the smoker can't relax since there is a second desire to satisfy. The smoker believes that smoking cigarettes can be the cherry of the cake however it's the small beast that has to be fed.

The truth is that the addiction to nicotine is never entirely comfortable. And it becomes more severe as you progress through life.

Smokers aren't the least stressed people in the world. The most stressed are business leaders who smoke in a chain constantly, cough and splutter and suffer from hypertension, and become increasingly angry. The cigarettes stop after this point, but only partially helping to ease the symptoms they've been suffering from.

Nicotine in cigarettes can affect your brain, which can lead to withdrawal symptoms whenever you attempt to stop. This is the opinion of the NIH (National Institute of Health). You could experience a range of negative side consequences when this happens that include anxiety, irritability as well as a severe desire for nicotine.

Unfortunately, many people are looking for the next puff as withdrawal symptoms begin to ease the pain caused by withdrawal.

The changes within the brain can create an addiction to nicotine since your body becomes accustomed to absorbing nicotine into your system. This then develops into an addiction that could be difficult to over come.

While it can take some time to realize how nicotine affects you adverse heart and lungs-related side effects are generally the first ones that a person who smokes can suffer.

In certain instances smokers smoke to ease the stress caused by other addictions like drinking. But The doctor. Paul Aveyard of the University of Oxford states that smoking cigarettes is creating stress instead. If you work in an environment where smoking breaks are allowed, then you are aware that smokers are more likely to take longer breaks and sometimes even walk out. Recent research also indicates smokers participate in patterns of inhalation-hold-release during smoking, which is more similar to those used in meditation than normal breathing. Smoking cigarettes and deep breathing control could be a major component of addiction (Wells 2012).

If you don't have a desire to smoke, there's no reason not to make short breaks in order to recharge oneself. In fact, you might not feel qualified to do this kind of self-care if you don't have an addiction to manage.

Another explanation could be that it is difficult to believe that we are smoking something fun by taking a puff. We tend to match our experiences with our expectations, so we could consider it as if we think that smoking is enjoyable, even if it actually increases our feeling of discontent and stress levels.

Smoking Improves Focus

Numerous studies have proven that nicotine may increase focus and concentration (making people who smoke feel awake). But there's more to cigarettes that just nicotine. The silent killer is comprised of around four thousand chemicals , over fifty of them are believed to be harmful in nature. These include carbon monoxide is commonly found in exhaust fumes from cars as well as butane in lighter fluids and, as an example arsenic and ammonia and methanol within rocket fuel.

In time, the build-up of these harmful chemicals could affect the brain, causing problems with memory and learning. Long-term smoking is linked to a decline in working memory and memory of the future, each of them required in everyday tasks, such as making an appointment or taking medications on time. They also have executive function that helps us organize our time focus on your current tasks and avoid distractions. These three functions support our daily ability to remember and comprehend and remember, without which it would be very difficult to be able to live independently.

Marshall Heffernan, Marshall Hamilton conducted a study back in 2016 to determine the synergistic effect that smoking cigarettes has on memory. in the Journal Frontiers in Psychiatry, these researchers from Northumbria University published their findings that people who smoke and drink regularly have more problems with their daily memory. In fact, they are more deficient that those who drink, but don't drink heavily or who drink heavily, but don't smoke. It is clear that, while smoking cigarettes may increase concentration in the short-term but the effect reverses in the in the long run - being a double-edged sword.

Always a smoker

If a person decides to stop smoking, cigarettes cravings are often the initial and longest-lasting withdrawal signs. Initially, these cravings can be intense however, they typically decrease as a person continues to go without smoking.

It is crucial to not only look not only stay away from the timeframe that these urges occur, as well as what steps you can adopt to counter the desire to smoke to overcome the cravings and avoid repeat.

Perhaps you've met an ex-smoker who says they'll always miss smoking, even though they've never had cigarettes for 20 years ago. This is a scary claim to make and yet they're in that position for a reason and it's something you could solve for yourself.

Smokers, the majority of us think that we are addicted to smoking however the reality is that we enjoy the sensation of relaxation when our bodies replenish their decreasing nicotine level. Nicotine withdrawal occurs when we stop smoking an cigarette. The physical urge to ease the pain is correlated to the activity we're engaged in the moment. It happens several times per day as our minds are conditioned into believing that smoking cigarettes is vital to having a fulfilling life over the course of.

Many famous individuals have managed to get over the pain of smoking and they've not turned back not once.

Barack Obama

The former president started smoking in his teens and then spoke about his addiction in an effort to live. In 2007 Obama said he would stop smoking tobacco on ABC. He ate Nicorette in order to prevent succumbing to the cravings that are triggered by the President's stress. He is aware that his battle against smoking continues. He signed an anti-smoking law in 2009 to stop the next generation from getting into smoking cigarettes.

Gisele Bundchen

As with other model women, Gisele was a smoker as way to keep her slim physique. The year 2003 was the time she quit her addiction in order to lead an ideal life for herself as well as her kids and became a role model for children. Bundchen states that when she made the decision to stop smoking she gained about 15 pounds, however she felt much more content with her healthier, new body.

Jennifer Aniston

The TV and film star was an avid chain smoker for a number of decades before beginning a cleanse in 2007. Aniston attributes her success to yoga. She is regularly active and eats a healthy diet to get rid of nicotine and caffeine.

Chapter 8: Why Does Smoking Seem So Difficult To Stop?

Nicotine is extremely addictive.

Smoking cigarettes is among the most difficult habits to eliminate. It is also common for users say that it's more difficult to quit the smoking habit than it is to quit the habit of crack.

A study from 2013 conducted carried out by researchers at an investigator from University of Massachusetts Medical School identified a specific group of neurons located at the midbrain's base within the interpeduncular nucleus which triggers anxiety and stress while observing an abstinence from nicotine. In this study, Andrew Tapper and his colleagues from the lab taught mice to become nicotine addicts. After they cut off nicotine, the mice began inexplicably shaking, trembling and shaking due to being wet and cold. While studying their brains mice, they found increased activity of neurons within a specific brain area known as the interpeduncular nuclear nucleus.

Opogenetics was the method used by researchers to created artificial stimulation of the same neurons using light. Subjects displayed behavior that resembled withdrawal from nicotine, regardless of whether or not the animal actually free of nicotine. In contrast, the effects of withdrawal from nicotine were cured by light treatment that decreased the activity in these neurons.

The interpeduncular nucleus receives signals from different areas of the brain that are involved in the usage and response to nicotine, and also anxiety-related sensations. The interpeduncular nucleus is surrounded with nicotinic acetylcholine receptors , which are target of nicotine's molecular structure. It is possible that the interpeduncular nuclear nucleus is linked to the withdrawal from certain types of addiction.

The results of a Duke University study showed that smokers who quit smoking might be wired to be successful in other areas that they face in life. The study published in the journal Neuropsychopharmacology in 2015 showed that enhanced functional connectivity in an

Insula-based Network is Associated with Improved Smoking Cessation Outcomes.

Researchers from Duke University discovered that those who had the ability to stop smoking had better co-ordination between the insula as well as the somatosensory cortex. This regulates our sensation of motor and touch. The improved contact was evident in smokers who quit smoking successfully from people who tried and did not succeed.

The insula is a large cerebral cortex region, typically considered to be the site of cravings and addictive impulses. The insula has been the focus of many different research into smoking cessation. According to the Duke study, researchers found that the stronger relationship between the insula and the somatosensory cortex was linked to smokers who have successfully stopped. Relapsed smokers had lesser interaction between these regions in the brain.

The insula plays a role when smokers want cigarettes. It can appear to light up when contemplating smoking while brain imaging. Other studies have revealed that smokers who suffer damage to the insula might suddenly lose their nicotine cravings, or even continue smoking cigarettes.

The Duke researchers looked at MRI scans from 85 people who were scanned for a month prior to when they attempted to stop smoking. Everyone who quit smoking cigarettes, and after 10 weeks, the researchers continued to monitor their findings. One participant were relapsed. Examining those brain scans taken by 44 smokers who had successfully quit The researchers discovered that, before quitting smoking they shared one thing in common: greater synergy between the insula as well as the somatosensory cortex.

In the near future, pharmaceuticals are likely to develop treatments that target specific areas of the brain to minimize harmful effects caused by withdrawal from nicotine and cravings. Meditation, mindfulness and neuro-feedback are all techniques for recovering that can be adapted to control brain activity to help smokers quit smoking.

The effects of withdrawal

The signs of withdrawal of the tobacco can start in the 20-30 minutes following the last time you used tobacco. It will also depend on your level of addiction. Other factors like the length of time you have been smoking and the amount of smoking carried out on a day to day basis can affect the severity of the symptoms.

Some symptoms consist of sweating and tingling feet and hands as well as insomnia, irritability and trouble concentrating as well as weight gain and depression. The withdrawal symptoms from nicotine usually manifest over a period of 2 to 3 days.

The brain's receptors for nicotine are the reason for cravings. As a result of your prior use of nicotine the receptors in your brain are increased. The messages received by receptors can encourage you to continue smoking. The absence of certain receptor signals can result in withdrawal symptoms.

However, they will begin to fade when you begin to ignore them. It is possible to see withdrawal symptoms disappearing within about two or four weeks. Certain people may endure a few months of withdrawal from nicotine.

Certain withdrawals from nicotine are preventable If we take the appropriate steps:

* Sore throat and dry mouth can be avoided with plenty of fluids chewing gum and drinking sugar-free lollipops.

* Deep breathing exercises aid in reducing headaches. Additionally, you can take non-prescription pain medication such as Advil as well as Tylenol.

If you are experiencing difficulties sleeping, you should turn off your devices at least 2 hours prior to your bedtime. Find other things to do such as reading, taking warm showers or listening to relaxing music instead.

* If you experience trouble focus or concentration, you should break for several minutes in the middle of your work.

Eat hard candy or carrots if you are feeling the urge to smoke.

Chapter 9: A Emotional Push

You can improve the health of your family members, friends employees, friends, and even your pets by not smoking. The harm of smoking cigarettes is evident to those you love.

Family members

If you have children at home, it is important to remember that smoking in their presence can increase the risk of asthma, ear infections as well as other breathing problems including bronchitis.

Children who are exposed to their parents smoke cigarettes are more likely develop into smokers later on in life too. In addition, being an adult doesn't shield anyone from the negative effects of smoking cigarettes. Smoke from secondhand cigarettes affects the lungs and heart of everyone within your home at risk, regardless of how many windows open or the number of fans you use.

Coworkers

Even if you're at work you're not smoking cigarettes Your colleagues could be affected. Smoking can affect your work effectiveness, as well as all the potential health risks associated with smoking. Asthma, heart disease, and weakened immune system will make you take more off days that a non-smoking coworker. A study found that smoking cigarettes cost companies an additional $5,816 annually (Berman, Crane, Seiber and Munur 2014)

Our Neighbors

Secondhand smoke is a source of more than 7000 chemicals. Many of them have been harmful and have been found that they cause cancer. Inhaling secondhand smokeor from a lit cigarette in the neighbor's house or from a smoke outside one's window has been proven to cause immediate adverse effects on people's cardiovascular system. In time smoking secondhand smoke can damage the lungs of a person and has been found increasing the likelihood of suffering from stroke up to 20-30.

Additional Research

In the year 2018, a study carried out by Kim, Ko, Kwon and Lee The results of which revealed that smoking secondhand cigarettes can increase the risk of cancer for those who have never smoked, especially breast and lung cancers particularly in women. The strictest implementation of smoking cessation programs must be promoted not just to reduce smoking, but also to limit secondhand smoking exposure.

Amer and his coworkers in the year 2018 published a study that looked at the effects of smoking secondhand on children. Nearly 3400 students in secondary and intermediate school located in Saudi Arabia were the subjects of the study. The most danger in exposure to smoking secondhand is associated with the smoking habits of the child. This is first caused through the parents (family structure) and then by close friends who smoke. The danger of exposure within the home was greatly elevated when combined with smoking cigarettes by the parents.

Chapter 10: Psychological Barriers

Smokers have daily challenges to quit smoking. Recognizing these obstacles is essential as they may be the only thing standing between you and stopping smoking.

The barriers are usually based upon misconceptions, and could be eliminated by recognizing the facts and preparing thoroughly.

Handling Stress

Many smokers are shocked find out that smoking increases tension!

It is normal to feel anxious and anxious (nicotine withdrawal) as the level of nicotine in your body fluctuates between cigarettes. In the course of the day, similar symptoms are common and can be eased by smoking another. It's not difficult to understand why smokers believe that they are comforted by cigarettes even though their smoking habits actually caused the issue first!

Smokers often smoke during the day to cope with stress in particular forms. While smoking reduces stress from withdrawals, smoking can not relieve certain types of stress, like fighting with your spouse, or a deadline stress.

The relief you get from smoking cigarettes is the result of taking breaks, not smoking the cigarette itself or even taking some deep breaths.

Many people feel regret or guilt for smoking. They are worried about the dangers to their health, which can also cause anxiety.

Nicotine can have a short-term calm effect, but is also an stimulant which triggers adrenaline as well as other chemicals that stimulate the heart rate, increases blood pressure and creates exuberance.

In the short run Quitting smoking can trigger anxiety, however anti-smoking medications will generally ease stress. Furthermore, studies have shown that even after quitting smokers who quit have less depression and are happier. The improved mental health of people is generally maintained for a long time following quitting.

Additionally, smoking cigarettes isn't a good solution to stress, and it can actually make things more difficult.

Weight Gain

The weight gain following stopping smoking is a primary issue for smokers of all ages and women, especially.

You're artificially from becoming overweight by smoking. When you quit smoking your body returns to its weight as if you'd never ever smoked.

The weight gain maximum in the first five years is 2.6 kilograms, even with the habit of smoking. This is less than the majority of smokers believe. Few are able to gain weight. A quarter of quitters gain weight or remain the same. Some quitters might gain more than the average.

The great news is that the huge benefit of quitting is far greater than the harm caused by any weight increase. It was found that in order to offset the health benefits that come with quitting the habit, you'll need to add 42 kilograms.

Your appearance can alter in many ways once you leave. The color of your skin improves and wrinkles will be less noticeable. You'll lose fingers and teeth due to those yellow stainings of tar. It's not like an ashtray any more.

Why do we gain weight?

The weight gain after stopping smoking is due in part to the stoppage of nicotine. Nicotine is a method to help keep weight off.

1. Nicotine reduces appetite. This is why you feel hungry for a few days after quitting smoking, which leads to eating more.
2. Nicotine can also boost metabolism and burns fat more effectively in the body. In the end, one could gain weight even if they consume the same quantity as they did before.

Can I avoid gaining weight?

Research has proven that trying to control your weight in a way that is too extreme when you're done with it usually fails and may also lower the chance of actually completing your quit. The best way to go about it is to follow healthy, low-fat, and low-fat eating habits keep exercising regularly and recognize that there's likely to be an rise in weight.

Crying

If you are a smoker is a habitual way of being able to have a certain amount of nicotine within your body. After quitting cravings start to arise because you are craving nicotine to your body. There are times when you may experience cravings for nicotine when you observe smokers or you're around other triggers.

In about an hour or so after you have smoked your last cigarette the cravings will begin. Each craving lasts for about 2 minutes, but it can seem like a lifetime! As time passes, cravings diminish and decrease and diminish.

Advertising

In a second theory, which was formulated in another theory by Eric Medneades, tobacco companies influence the customers they are targeting through playing with their needs. For instance, during the 1950's, women across the USA were not smoking. However, a corporation saw that women had begun to struggle for their rights and decided to incorporate smoking into the scene. They depicted women smoking cigarettes and enjoying their new freedom. There was an abrupt increase in the number of women smoking cigarettes in the US. This is a counterproductive placebo effect.

It is essential to avoid falling into the trap of these ads and strive to be rational when we see them. Consider your goals. Imagine yourself reaching it. Consider whether this product is going assist me in becoming an improved version of myself? If not, then you should get rid of it.

Chapter 11: What's The Science Behind Bad Habits

It's not easy to let go of routines. We've all experienced this as we've stumbled across times when we've missed our diet change, or felt the constant urge to keep our Twitter feed updated instead of working on a task due to a deadline. In the present, choosing to act differently when stressed is difficult, particularly when you're surrounded by modern conveniences such as tobacco additives, processed sugar and endless lists of tasks.

Our brains are constantly bombarded with stimuli created to induce us to want to consume food. This type of stimulus can be a sabotage to the reward-based learning mechanism in our brains which was initially designed to help us survive. In simple terms, learning based on reward requires an initial trigger (such such as hunger) and is followed by an the action (eating foods) as well as reward (feeling satisfied). We'd like to focus on the positive things, and less negative ones.

Every time we light cigarettes or eat a cake, or browse our newsfeed when you're feeling depressed, these three parts of trigger, behavior and reward, appear. The learning process is strengthened each time we reach to find something to relax ourselves until it becomes effortless. Habits are built this way.

What's the reason we can't observe and then agree to create new habits for ourselves? In spite of the fact research at Yale have demonstrated that prefrontal cortex (its function is usually related to the ability to control oneself) can be the very first brain to shut down when confronted with stimuli such as stress, the concept that self-control is a good thing has been adduced for a long time. We've all experienced this in some way that when we're angry or exhausted and stressed, we're more likely shout at a loved one or go to the refrigerator regardless of how many times we rebuke the behavior each time we do it.

Brains can be wired to take on new behaviors. Let's experiment:

1. Record your behavior patterns: Learning that is reward-driven is based by, well, rewards and not the behaviour itself. That

is, the way that behavior has rewarded the chance of repeating that behavior later on.

2. Be aware of the different sensations: Be aware of the various sensations you experience while smoking -is it a pleasant smell and taste like? It is frequently observed that the same thing occurs time and time again when people realize that smoking isn't very pleasing for their senses.

3. Find innovative ways to reward yourself. last step to create a permanent significant change in behavior is to identify an objective or a dream that is healthier as compared to the present one. The brain is still looking for greater value and a better bargain. Janes and colleagues in the year 2019 conducted research to determine the effects that mindfulness has on smokers' signals. The results revealed that smokers also learned how to control their default mode system which in turn reduces smokingthe same brain system is activated over time by signals from smoking and chocolate cravings as well as calmness among professional meditators.

Imagine you're trying to kick a bad habit, like smoking, binge eating, or a sense of anxiety. What if instead, you were to pursue your curiosity about the addiction to create a new habit instead of just doing what you want to smoke or consume chips of potato to fight the negative emotions?

The purpose behind the reward is different from the tangible: The feeling of interest is stronger than the desire. It allows us to explore and not lulling us in a frenzied search to consume. The pursuit of curiosity is typically better than self-blame and reflection. They often coincide with patterns that we would like to investigate.

Chapter 12: What Can I Stop Smoking

Although some smokers are successful at quitting smoking cold turkey, the majority of people opt for a customized plan to monitor their own progress. A successful strategy for quitting addresses the short-term issue as well as the long-term aim of staying clear of the possibility of relapse. It must be tailored to meet your individual requirements and smoking habits as well.

Consider thinking about the type or smoker you're and which circumstances in your life trigger smoking a cigarette and why. This will assist you in determining what strategies, methods, or methods could provide the most benefit to you.

Am I a heavy smoker?

Is there a specific spot where I'm a fan of smoking at?

Should I be smoking when I'm stressed? Social gathering? Office?

Utilize the S.T.A.R.T method to start your smoking program.

S = Set a date to quit

Select a time within fourteen days from now to ensure you'll have enough time to plan your day without sacrificing your drive. If you smoke a lot at work, you should make the quit plan for weekends, so you've the opportunity to make the necessary adjustments to the change.

T = Inform your family as well as your friends, family, and coworkers.

Inform your family and friends about your plans and let them know that you're looking for their help and support to stop smoking. Find a quit-mate who's also looking to quit smoking. It is important to support each other in the tough times

A= Be Prepared for the Upcoming Challenge

The majority of smokers who smoke do it in the initial three months. Prepare yourself for the coming issues like nicotine withdrawal and cravings for cigarettes. This will assist you in making it through

R = Get rid of all tobacco/smoking related products

Take out all your cigarettes and lighters, ashtrays, lighters and matches you've got. Cleanse the clothes you wear and clean anything that smells of smoke. Cleanse your car with an aroma-laden detergent. You can also make use of a softener for your clothes. Steam your carpet, as well as furniture.

T = Speak with your doctor

Your doctor may prescribe medication to ease the withdrawal symptoms. If you don't have access to an expert. You can visit the local pharmacy to purchase various items on the market, like nicotine patches, lozenges and gum

The most important thing your self can accomplish is identify what triggers you to desire to smoke, such as particular situations such as habits, emotions, and other people.

A journal of your cravings can aid in focusing on the reasons behind your addiction and your trends. Keep track of your cigarettes for approximately an entire week before the date you decide to quit. Recall the times when you long to smoke a cigarette each day and ask yourself these following questions:

When did the craving begin?

On a scale from 1-10, how severe were the cravings?

What was you doing at the time it happened?

Did you have a relationship with someone?

What were your feelings emotionally?

What did you feel like after you smoked?

Tips for avoiding common Triggers

Alcohol:

The majority of those who drink tend to smoke regularly. Consider shifting your drinking habits towards non-alcoholic beverages or drinking only in places that prohibit smoking inside. Think about snacking on nuts or drinking a straw as an alternative.

Smoking Buddies:

If your family, friends and colleagues smoke around you, quitting or avoiding relapse could be more difficult. Make a decision about quitting so that everyone knows and avoid smoking when you're driving or while taking a break for coffee. Find people who aren't smokers at your workplace to share breaks with you, or discover an activity that is new such as walking.

Meals

The end of a meal is a time to light up for some smokers, and the idea of giving it up may be overwhelming. After a meal it is possible to replace the meal with something different, such as an apple slice or a nutritious cookie or chocolate square or a piece or a chewing gum substitute.

Consistency is key.

The ability to stick to your goals is an important thing, but staying on the path for the long haul is the tough part. An understanding of the factors that is behind these attempts is required for determining effective ways to boost the number of attempts to quit. In this regard the motivation to quit is a significant factor. Simple evaluations of motivation for stopping at a certain moment in time, and more nuanced ratings of motivation, desire and faith were found to be extremely predictors of efforts to quit over the next few months.

In a study carried out by Perski along with her colleagues of University College London, a cross-sectional study was carried out to determine the relation between motivation to quit and the consistency of. This study involved 16,657 participants that were examined from 2012 until 2017. Smokers were asked about their serious desire to quit smoking in the last year, and then they were asked two questions on motivation to quit smoking (current motivation) and to keep going (continuous motivation). The participants had at least one attempt to stop smoking during the previous year. Together with the existing motivation to quit, and the constant motivation to quit individually, and in conjunction with both models adapting to socio-demographic factors and an indicator of nicotine dependence was regressed by logistic models.

The results of the study revealed that the persistence of motivation to quit smoking substantially increases the likelihood of the effort to quit smoking, even if it is not a present motivation.

Chapter 13: What Brought You To Smoking?

I'm not sure!

I'm not able think for you And who told me I had to be able to do everything in this book?

Do a bit of work on the project yourself.

You're in trouble. I'll tell you the truth I'll do to understand your thoughts.

It was a difficult moment within your personal life. Numerous events physically raged against you and weakened you. It was like being a frog out of water and could not find a way to soothe your troubled soul.

You've seen the large words The style, I could write!

You did it just right from the beginning. Gotcha!

What? I didn't get it. Isn't that what you were looking for when you started smoking cigarettes?

Oh, that's a disappointment... Go back three squares in case my claim does not convince you, or go forward five squares if the statement corresponds to.

I'm trying to be nice to you. If you aren't happy with my suggestion, take an instant, place the tablet or book in your lap (you most likely lie down now) and shut your eyes for one second.

Beware! Every person who reads this has confirmed my claim can skip this section and move on to the next chapter. I am forced to remain here to assist people who are confused. We are a fantastic team here. No one is left behind by their partner.

Have you thought of my statements for just a second? Are you in agreement with my assertion? Do you have any doubts? Can you think of other motive?

I'm not trying to hurry you, but other people have made progress.

Did you move? You made it because of curiosity? To show your rebellious side? to make you feel more cool?

This isn't the case. You have to go deeper. Don't be scared I'm here. Follow me.

Answer these questions in a few minutes: Would you leap off an rock? Would you be able to jump off a plane with no parachute? Would you smash the thumb of your hand with a large hammer? It's not possible! Are you aware of the reason? Because, if you were stupid, you'd either die , or suffer excessively for no reason whatsoever.

You first smoked cigarettes due to the fact that you were feeling not comfortable at the moment and you felt that you had to take a step forward. Something that could provide the needed boost. Defying death. In that moment, you made the decision that the world wasn't so great and it was the time to feel alive, unbreakable. You wanted to prove to you and your friends (unfortunately) that no fear could ever stop you and that you were ready for the end of your life.

Did you find it too direct? Dude I've been there during this time, so I can't trust you.

If you're really determined to quit smoking or, more precisely, to fight death, you must get your cards out and begin living your life to the fullest.

I believe you've aligned yourself with me. Let's move on into the new chapter.

Do not worry, I assured that you would have fun reading this book and I promise you'll have fun too however, this painful issue was a must be addressed. Be aware that when you don't touch your bottom you will not be able to taste the top.

This is the foundation of Tao as a concept in Eastern tradition and also in culture!

Sometimes I'm amazed by how well-educated I am! I love it!

Why do you continue to smoke?

We're back. The dearest friend of ours has conquered his doubts and is here with us once more.

I'll share a new insight. A lot people have read through the preceding chapter, even though you were in agreement with me on my point. Reason?

Then, you've paid for the entire book, in case you happen to fail to read one or two pages.

What is right is what is right!

Let's get moving.

After I've caught your attention, and I'm linked to your brain I'm able to manipulate it in any way I like. Are you prepared?

One... two... three.

Stop smoking! Stop right now! It's a good time to need to quit smoking right now!

Thanks for all your kind words. My sole goal was to get you to stop smoking, while having fun and I'm certain I did it.

The book comes to an end here.

I'd like to receive a huge applause!

Are you still reading?

I must admit that the urge to end the book in this manner was strong. It could have been fantastic.

The true essence. If it had been done this way, it would have been a better way to understand the whole idea.

An original text that could have convinced you that you have the option of quitting anytime.

It's a stroke of genius! They'd have mentioned me across all social media platforms and on TV shows. Perhaps I'd been invited to "The Ellen DeGeneres Show"The book that has changed the lives of many people. In the newspaper, it is "the novel of revelations from the past century. It sticks in your head and causes you to stop smoking cigarettes."

Humanity, unfortunately, is extremely complicated. It's never enough.

You'd be ridiculed for not writing at minimum at least 10 or 11 pages therefore, despite my own ego, I must set aside my self-importance and continue writing for you.

Where are we now?

Do you ever try to stop between the last chapter and the current one?

Did you get a snap out of it?

If you don't reply then you've been sloppy You're the man! You're the one!! You have mastered the essentials of the book and then quit on your own since you recognized that living is truly beautiful and that defying death is not a good thing.

If you're still reading instead ....

Let's continue.

Answer this question. Why do you continue to smoke?

If you're willing I'll provide you with the solution.

Since you enjoy the taste. Ah...how enjoyable you can smoke.

Do you give it up because of who? Do you wish to smoke cigarettes in your morning after coffee or breakfast?

or the smoke after lunch or after a sex? What would you do to sacrifice this incredible pleasure? What would you exchange it for? What else could you do to please you in the same manner?

Okay! I'll admit that you've got plenty of work ahead of your life. Take a look at yourself, now I must spend a lot of time creating and trying to persuade you, or even to help you break those beliefs that you have.

However, is it possible that you don't know the assertions you make (yes I'm sure they're mine, however I'm reminding you that I'm an ex-smoker. I read a lot of books, and I've was able to read your mind) aren't true?

They result from an untrue, deviant notion that you made yourself to be invincible. Not when you took the first cigarette, which was the battle with death, and that in that moment you demonstrated to your self that you were invincible, but rather by smoking the second one, after that the third, the fourth , and so on.

As you continued to smoke, you believed that it was beneficial for you. You felt cool, relaxed and felt like you were part of a community. Smokers. The truth is in your eyes.

You're indestructible. You're indestructible! Dear friend, you're there, and you've proven it at numerous other times. You're very resilient and unstoppable, you just need to keep in mind all the challenges that you've faced throughout your life and all the battles you've fought and the obstacles you've faced. I'd like to see others take your shoes, they could have collapsed, but you emerged the victor, since you're an ace. You're a true warrior.

It's time to take your claws and show the world what you can do take on the smoking habit.

I'm confident that there's nothing more beautiful than riding a bike with your family or friends and declaring, "I quit smoking."

They'll all stare at your face with eyes full of amazement, as if you'd just won the battle between two worlds. Wow! How did you manage that? (Here you need to be honest and confess that you've done it).

I have read my book, but because the credit was largely yours, he exaggerates excites, and even creates.

You're due!

However, for me, I think it's the right time to end the parenthesis!)

Define the word "sloth.

Listen to me because this may be the pivotal moment.

Sloth is actually an of seven vices that are deadly, so imagine how vital it is. I'll provide the complete definition on Wikipedia I'm talking about that's not pizzas and figs.

Acedia, or sloth, is a reluctance to operate as a result of boredom and indifference. The origin of the classical etymology is derived from word from the Greek the

Greek words a (alpha privative, meaning without) and kedos (means cure) that is synonymous with indolence. It is derived from it's Latin Vulgar acedia.

In the ancient world of Greece the term acedia (akedia) was a reference to an inert condition of not feeling suffering and concern, indifference, and consequently sadness and sadness. The word was used once more in the Middle Ages, as a notion of moral theology to refer to the melancholic trance and inertia of people who had a contemplative pursuits. Thomas Aquinas defined it as the "sadness of divine goodness" that is capable of causing an inertia when it comes to acting on in the name of God's good.

The meaning of the word is closely linked to that of boredom. both share the same basic state that is governed by the contemplative lifestyle Both are the state of happiness and , if you think about it, not in the need.

I'm sure you know the meaning of acedia. we'd have missed the definition, but it was to clarify the meaning for all readers.

Now , the question is.

The process.

Keep your eyes on the prize. You've said you'd love to run for exercise on Monday. That's the aim. Exercise is beneficial for your health everyone is aware of that. Everyday you will are likely to see people out running on the streets But be aware of one important thing.

Take the time to think about and think about what you saw around your during Christmas Day last year, most likely between 10am and 6pm.

Are you remembering? Let me assist you. I'm sure that you've said it:

"Who is running at night on Christmas Day? It's likely to be a solo runner.

Now that I've written the sentence, I'm writing was written using Roman to give it the correct accent, perhaps you read it in your own dialect. I believe the idea did come to you in the end.

The person who ran at 10:30 am Christmas Day sounded strange to you. So, I'd like to let you know that you're the wrong person!

The person running was human who runs out of desire, and to feel happy about himself. He is an intelligent egoist. Maybe his wife had told him:

"But you're not going to go out today. When it's Christmas, will you be out for a run? Keep here for an hour and I'll make sure you're smile! Would you rather run rather than be here with me, along with your children, and grandparents, and your brother-in law and your mother-in-law ...?"

Yes, it is. He is a runner and prefers to run at the same time. There is no time for celebrations. He has to run because when he's done, he'll feel at ease with himself and will be ready to show love to his neighbors.

This is a simple statement and I can assure you that it is.

The passion will be revealed to you in the future. Take a moment to think about it, consider an idea you had in your head and how it came into being.

At first, you just experimented and enjoyed it so much that you decided to keep going without anyone convincing or insisting on your doing it. Why not give it a go?

You're probably thinking what's the procedure? How fast I was getting there.

Let's revisit the race on Monday. In addition to running, I'd suggest the benefits of walking at a high speed You're definitely out of condition and smoke (I am not a fan of smoking and I'm sick of it).

It's Monday, and, as if by chance you've forgotten all the positive intentions and are at the beginning stage,

What should you do? Follow my steps attentively.

The first step is to create an evening reminder on your mobile with the reminder to dress in your tracksuit and sneakers.

With the help of the reminder, make sure you have your tracksuit and your shoes near your bed. In the evening, before going to the bed.

The first thing you do when you get up the first thing to do is take off your tracksuit and shoes in the closet. Once you've completed this simple procedure, you can return to your normal routine.

Repeat this process every day for 10 consecutive weeks.

All clear so far? I'm sure you're not able to say that I'm dumb, but try asking yourself if you're evident so far.

At night, with the memo, you make small things that you need to take running , and the next morning, you return them. It's easy, isn't it?

Let's begin. The tenth day is when you repeat the same procedure but this time , you put on the suit and shoes at the beginning of the day and after that you get dressed by carefully arranging your clothing.

Well, that's it! It's time to begin your incredible journey as non-professional athlete.

By following my advice according to the exact letter If you follow my instructions to the letter, you'll achieve two wonderful outcomes. The first is that you've finally incorporated the process of getting ready for running into your day-to-day routine.

After two weeks , it is normal to take this and things will be simpler now.

The other amazing thing you'll have accomplished is feeling as if you're an idiot for performing these things without running. Do you believe? after two weeks, maybe you could walk out on the streets and go for a the 10 minutes walk?

You'll be amazed and soon you'll be walking every day, running, stretching. You'll likely have already stopped smoking. This technique can apply to any goals you'd like to accomplish and the best part is that I didn't come up with this method, therefore it's not a flimsy idea. If you'd like to learn more about this enduring mental method, I recommend you take the time to look up YouTube in search of "Marco Montemagno" my mentor. He is a digital entrepreneur and social motivational expert.

There are a variety of videos on many subjects and some of them are focused on motivation. In this video, he goes over this method of success to include into our lives automatic mechanisms that allow us to reach our objectives while reducing the work.

Keep your promises.

A child comes up to the father of his friend and inquires:

"Daddy Where do us come from?

The father responds:

"We are the descendents from Adam as well as Eve."

Son: "But mom said we are monkeys!"

Father: "Your mother's family is different."

You're aware

We're ready.

We're kidding, we have two more points to discuss and then you'll be able to stop smoking.

As of now, you've realized that life is wonderful and should not be wasted. If you are required to embark on the new chapter but do not feel the enthusiasm, you need to design simple and simple actions in your everyday life to allow the journey to be easier and more efficient The passion will begin to flow.

In this moment, I'd like to talk with you about the most delicate topic the issue of convictions.

You smoke, sure it's a habit But at the core of it all are false beliefs that don't let you quit smoking due to them being so deeply embedded within you that you are unable to believe that they result from an incorrect mental process.

If we don't take them out in tandem, you'll never be capable of quitting smoking.

This time I'd like to provide you with the definition, even from Wikipedia Here is the definition:

"conviction s. f. [from lat. tardo convictio - onis, remade on part. conviction]. Conviction - Believing; conviction or moral certainty especially when acquired through overpowering doubts and contradicting motives to unite, impart the impression of acquiring the confidence. shake an shake a. and have a full of a deep, unshakeable and rooted conviction. Be unshakeable in one's own. and talk with conviction. The thing that makes one is persuaded, convinced, or convinced."

Beautiful, isn't it? These few sentences is in a way the reason you're not able to quit smoking quickly.

I'll note some notes to refresh your thoughts:

If I stop smoking, I'll be fatter.

If I quit smoking I'm unable to stay calm in situations of stress...

If I stop smoking, I'm not attractive.

If I quit smoking, I can't concentrate...

If I stop smoking cigarettes, I won't be able to socialize with other people.

If you are able to imagine another reason to take note of it and note it down. It's the one keeping you from your goals the most. This isn't a joke. It's time to get involved too.

Grab a piece of paper and note down every reason you smoke.

Advice. When you record it in your cell phone's memo app, you may be tempted to lose it.

It's very well. Now, you're faced with the list of myths which will make you put that cigarette in your mouth.

You can destroy your convictions then you're finished! I can hear you already. Okay, fine, and If it were that easy I wouldn't even consider buying the book. I'm not sure what to do. Forint, I need you to assist me!

Tell me your secrets. How did you stop smoking cigarettes? What mysterious and mysterious ancient ritual did you follow to stop smoking?

Relieve yourself, relax! I'll be there.

At this point, I'm extremely concerned. If I said that it was simple to quit smoking, and that you could use the next method to stop smoking, it would likely disappoint you.

But howdo I get there? If it's that easy to quit, then why wouldn't I quit earlier and for myself? Are I a fool?

There's no way you're an fool. There's no way! You don't even know how to go about it.

Did you remember when you first learned to use a bicycle?

It seems like I'm in the wrong path here. I don't want to be anyone among the readers who doesn't have the ability to cycle. Let me tell you something is for those who aren't able to ride a bike and smoke, they can still smoke and I'd advise them to give up.

Was I too harsh? Are you aware of the reasons why you can't use a bicycle? I'm not going to reveal it this moment. You'll have to wait until the new edition of my book "Learning the art of riding a bicycle with a smile" is out.

Let's take a ride on the bicycle. When you were a kid, you were motivated by curiosity. It was initially difficult and you were unable to keep your balance and fall, but then you laughed.

What an amazing depth of thought! I'm awestruck at my own abilities.

There weren't any negative convictions. Fear of injury and creating a bad impression fears of accidents and fear of the judgement of those in your vicinity.

This is why you hopped on your bike and tried , and tried, and failed to keep your balance and pedal.

Your views. In this moment, I'd even say they are fears.

Let's eliminate these fears, and you'll quit smoking.

A renowned savant of human intelligence can come to your rescue. Someone who's studied the subject, one that you can trust, when he publishes a book, you'll purchase it without looking at it. The legendary Vincent Fanelli, author of several books, such as "The Quantum Mind".

A book that I highly recommend reading for its informational content that is detective-like, and on how you can change your perspective and focus on your universe.

Because of the application of the concepts that are the foundation of this book, I could quit smoking cigarettes easily.

Do you still find the word to cause you anxiety? Do you want me to not to speak about it?

Okay! I was able to stop with immense difficulty and intense fatigue. In any case, to fact, make this a reference whenever someone asks you what you did to ended your journey.

Let's get our attention now. I'll show you how to overcome your fears about smoking cigarettes.

Follow my steps step-by-step or you'll be required to purchase The book "The Mind When You Smoke".

I'll try to summarise the process for you in just a few phrases and you need to believe me.

I'm ready.

The first thing that you need to do is get out of the house right now, with your book in your hand . Then you need to purchase something small that you love, which you can carry in your hands and wear whenever you like without raising suspicions regarding how you'll make use of it over a long period of time. I would suggest objects like rings, bracelets or pendant. You could also purchase pen, but the three above are the most practical.

Do not spend a lot of money on these, Chinese products are fine as well. It'll be a useful item at first and you'll use it often, and then you can remove it at any time.

Here , you can pick the item you want to purchase.

When you've finished with the thing you need set it aside.

The memo is open and look at the list of thoughts and fears that you wrote on your mobile phone. Take a look at the first entry.

You can now lie down or sit however you want and do not let anyone disturb your attention in any manner. I'll offer you some tips. Use this method in the event that you're on your own.

Keep your eyes open, and you will see two distinct areas that are in front of your eyes, one to the left and another to the right of your eye. To grasp this, you have to place yourself in such that you are able to let your eyes open and look at the wall in the front of you. It doesn't matter what color or the photos which are displayed.

Relax your eyes, close them and breathe deeply for five minutes.

Imagine a task that's simple for you. I've used the example of driving my car around my home. You must pick the car that best represents you, for instance, going out for drinks at the bar.

My plan is to walk up to my car, get the keys from my pocket, put them in the car, shut the door, turn on the engine and drive without crying. I walk around the block and then park the car again.

That's it! A task that I could quickly complete.

You can try it.

The scene you've created display it on the right part of the wall the direction of your eyes like an art piece, a television or a screen.

Once you've imagined it then pay attention to the details. Then, answer these questions:

How is the size?

What shape is it made of?

How brilliant is it?

Are the colors crisp?

Are there words, sounds or sounds?

If you were able to be able to touch it, how do you think it would feel like?

This is crucial because it allows you to discover the ways your brain process the positive images you have.

Focus instead on your final goal. Stop smoking.

Imagine that you're about to take a puff put your hands in your pocket, and instead of cigarettes, you discover the item you purchased (the bracelet, the ring and so on.) You put it in your hands, gaze at it and be happy as you feel satisfied that you have quit smoking. You're so glad that you touch the object and lift it into the air like an enormous cup. You feel like you're a winner. You take the object out of the pocket of your bag, and take three large breaths and enjoy the fresh, pure air that flows into your lungs. You then go out to sing your favourite tune.

Once you've made this representation, look it up on your left wall. Then analyse it by answering the questions above.

How large is it?

What shape does it take?

How brilliant is it?
Are the colors crisp?
Are there words, sounds or sounds?
If you were able to be able to touch it, how do you think it would feel like?
Most likely, your interpretation will likely to differ than what you imagined as an action is easy to perform.
Then, you can you can rework the depiction of stopping smoking on the right edge of the wall to make it exact to the initial depiction. Make sure to not interfere in the main content however, focus on the specifics. To help you comprehend the situation, imagine that there are two TVs in your face and you must set the second one up by watching the first.
To better understand the meaning of a representation, for instance, if the first representation was an oval shape, and the second, which was about quitting smoking , was contained within an oval, it is necessary to recreate it inside a rectangleof the same dimensions. The colors have to be the same as the original

representation, as well as the sound and tactile aspect.

In short, you will need to modify this second representation to match the first.

If you've succeeded as I am certain that you have, we can go to the next step.

I would recommend it. If you can complete all the steps in a single day, great however if you are on a an extremely tight schedule, you could complete the different actions in 2 days. Be careful not to allow too long between each step to the next due to the many ideas you've written down, you risk missing the earlier steps and dissatisfying the end result.

Step 2

Find the list that is complete with your beliefs that you have written down.

There's the booze-smoker. She's the one who's not going to let you stop smoking cigarettes. Don't be mad at her!

I'm repeating my own thoughts because it's essential to the effectiveness of the technique. You'll need to repeat each false belief that you find in the list.

To help you comprehend all the steps, I'll give an example.

If you've done a little practice, it can take about five minutes for each conviction. Don't be rushed.

However, make sure you take all the time you require to be able to focus on any of the below
representation.

We must perform in reverse, and we need to dismantle the beliefs you hold, so we move in this manner.

I'm trying to dispel the notion that if I quit smoking, I'll gain weight.

Excellently. Always calm in front of the wall. Five deep breaths, and you're ready to start.

I must visualize on the left side of the wall, make sure I'm not saying left, a real-life incident that occurred to me or could occur to me, but very uncertain and uncertain.

For instance, as I'm getting ready to leave for work, and the forecast says it will not be raining for the next four hours but the sky doesn't promise anything positive. I'm in a quandary whether to bring the uncomfortable umbrella or pay attention to the forecast.

The image of this question will be muffled, smoky and blurred. I'll be able to see me with my eyes pointing to the sky, enticed by my head. I can see myself as if blurred. The entire image is the black-and-white. There's an awful amount of haze over me. The entire scene is projected in an old cathode-ray tube-based television that was made in the 70s.

Here's an illustration of how your representative sample should be utilized to help create the sense of uncertainty and doubt.

Create your own image as you would like it to appear, but the most important thing is that you have a solid doubt about it.

the image is not clearly identified and confusing.

Once you've completed this, fix the image to your left side. You must create a skewed image of yourself becoming fat once you stop smoking.

It should be fun, almost tacky and it should bring you a smile. However, you must imagine it in the same smoky, distorted contours, using the same scents, with the exact sensation, and placed in the same shape (remember? television, image projector) using which you made an image that posed doubt.

Now, place this on your right wall.

Now, you can move your thoughts the image of your fattening from the right toward the other side. This will make the doubtful image disappear.

As you can see, you have just one picture on the left on your wall. The right side should be filled with another image of you who have quit smoking , and haven't gained an ounce of weight. In fact, you're looking great looking happy and smiling. Be aware that this time, you'll need to construct it with the same qualities "of the way that's simple for you" therefore, the identical colors, similar smells and the same form of projection, and the list goes on. Easy, right?

I guarantee you that it requires a lot more words to describe it than be able to comprehend it.

Let me provide you with an overview of the following:

Create a visual image of an event that is easy to understand...

Create a depiction of a real doubt

To dispel negative beliefs, it casts uncertainty on left side and negative beliefs on the right

Transfer the negative sideboard to the left and then fill the right side with an image of the sideboard that you would like to take down.

Repeat this process for each of the items in the list you've made.

Take some time off. It's a bit tense.

I was acquainted with a woman who was beautiful in her body, but a terrible face. She was an balaclava model.

His husband says: "Why don't you ever let me know when you're having an orgasm? "The spouse: "Because when you do you're away from home."

When I was a kid, my parents took me to a group of children who were so poor that at the beach instead of castles we constructed sand-built houses.

I'm ready to smoke I'm going to all over Florence to look for an Tuscan.

To stop smoking, all you have to do is stop buying cigarettes. To stop drinking, you simply have to learn to swim.

He will ask you following an intercourse: "Miss, do you smoke?". "Smoking is not a good idea however it's hot! ".

"I'm trying to stop smoking." "Have you ever tried candy?". "Yes but they don't flash! ".

Okay I think we've relaxed enough.

Conclusions

This approach will address the root issue, you now have the tools needed and the path to redemption could be more accessible than you think even if you've struggled for years, as me, when you have put your heart into something, there's no reason why you're not able to achieve it Perhaps you wanted to know how or something that could inspire you. Now you know my story and how I achieved it.

This structure is solid and I'm sure it can work for you with the same effectiveness it has worked for my colleagues and me. Let yourself unleash your full potential by using it.

Addictions are only powerful as long as they are allowed to be. It is difficult to recognize when you're hooked on something. They are similar to creatures in our minds and we believe that they are more powerful than the things we can handle however this is not by any way true. It isn't just possible , but is also not as difficult as you believed when you understand how to handle the issues.

Give the credit due to your brain and then use it to your advantage, and work with it. It will be a great experience. Living a life free of chains of harmful routines is a great way to lead, but only those who have walked through the abyss and emerged from it in good health will be able to appreciate.

I am here to help you. extended to assist you and you're not alone and you are not the only one dealing with it. It isn't a matter of the reason we fell into it the most important thing is that we get on our feet. When you're done, you'll have a boost of self-esteem that is well earned, which is an incredible feeling. I know this because once I crossed the line and was on"the "free" side, I couldn't believe it was that easy to do, all I needed was the right map Now you've got the map.

It's an ongoing commitment, no matter if you have a slight sense of nostalgia and you want to smoke, or whatever comes up in your circumstance Do yourself a favor, and don't take that chance, you've been into the trap once earlier and there is no guarantee that you will never repeat the mistake and is not worth the risk.

I'd like to request you to now help me in spreading the word to those who need it. You can assist me by writing reviewing the book and sending this book out to anyone you know who is willing to read it, and make money from it.

I truly wish you the best in your endeavor, and be prepared with determination and strength.

Holly Father, as this line is read, shower your blessings on the person taking them in, and provide them with a light to their path and clear direction to remain on the right path in their journey. Keep the fire of inspiration that is burning in their hearts always burning vibrant and powerful, and remove temptations during the tough times and allow them to develop every day, and let them explore and revel in the wonderful things life offers them. Amen.

www.ingramcontent.com/pod-product-compliance
Lightning Source LLC
Chambersburg PA
CBHW071124130526
44590CB00056B/1882